THE JANE AUSTEN DIET

AUSTEN'S SECRETS TO FOOD, HEALTH, AND INCANDESCENT HAPPINESS

JANE AUSTEN AND BRYAN KOZLOWSKI

TURNER PUBLISHING COMPANY

Turner Publishing Company
Nashville, Tennessee
www.turnerpublishing.com

Cover design: Kerri Resnick
Book design: Tim Holtz

Library of Congress Cataloging-in-Publication Data

Names: Austen, Jane, 1775-1817, author. | Kozlowski, Bryan, author.
Title: The Jane Austen diet : Austen's secrets to health, food, and
   incandescent happiness / Jane Austen and Bryan Kozlowski.
Description: Nashville, Tennessee : Turner Publishing Company, 2019. |
   Identifiers: LCCN 2018021216 (print) | LCCN 2018022718 (ebook) | ISBN
   9781684422135 (epub) | ISBN 9781684422111 (hardback) |
   ISBN 9781684422128 (pbk.)
Subjects: LCSH: Health. | Nutrition. | Exercise. | Mind and body. |
   Self-care, Health.
Classification: LCC RA776 (ebook) | LCC RA776 .A85 2019 (print) | DDC
   613.2--dc23
LC record available at https://lccn.loc.gov/2018021216

9781684422128 Paperback
9781684422111 Hardcover

Printed in the United States of America
17 18 19 20 10 9 8 7 6 5 4 3 2 1

To my extraordinary parents,
Andy and Faith, with,
as Jane would say,
"a hundred thousand million kisses."

"One hears sometimes of a child
being 'the picture of health;' now
Emma always gives me the idea of
being the complete picture of
grown-up health. She is loveliness
itself. Mr. Knightley, is not she?"

—Emma

CONTENTS

"How I wish I lived in a Jane Austen novel!"

—Dodie Smith

PROLOGUE

"A BEGINNING IS MADE"

What can Jane Austen teach us about health? An English spinster from the 1800s sitting snugly beside a dish of tea and crumpets: the image doesn't exactly scream food-and-fitness guru for the twenty-first century. Too modest to even include a kissing scene in her *romance* novels, how could she possibly understand the complicated body, beauty, and weight-loss battles we face today? More to the point, did Jane Austen ever diet? A diet of what, pray? Plum pudding and port wine?

These were the questions buzzing through my brain in 2016: the year Austen revealed her extraordinary answers. Though it happened, as Jane herself would admit, "by a most fortunate chance." Two types of books had plonked themselves on my nightstand that year: the latest health and wellness books (for serious reading) and Jane Austen's novels (for fun). Both arrived for no other reason than pure vanity. My thirtieth birthday was fast approaching and I had a third-life crisis on my hands. To use a more Regency-appropriate metaphor, I was losing the "bloom of youth." Everything I took for granted in my early twenties—naturally high energy levels, the ability to eat anything without consequences, the genetically slim physique I *thought* was my cosmic birthright—was disappearing, and I wanted it back. The health books were there to make that happen. Austen was simply there, as any self-respecting Anglophile will tell you, to provide moral support for the journey. She ended up providing so much more.

I noticed it almost immediately—that is, after rubbing my eyes from the shock. There were details in *Pride and Prejudice* and *Sense and Sensibility* that paralleled, almost exactly, the latest "discoveries" in the most modern dieting books available. In one moment I would read about the newest scientific research on eating, exercise, and holistic living and then realize moments later that Jane had said the same thing (albeit with more elegance and wit) over two hundred years ago. It happened too frequently to be a fluke. The more I read, the more Austen was amazingly rubbing shoulders with the brightest minds in health, food, and total-body wellness three centuries ahead of her time.

To quote Lydia Bennet, "I was ready to die of laughter." This was not the Jane Austen I thought I knew. *My* Austen wrote Regency romance novels, not diet books. She's the woman who ruins love lives with impossible, Darcy-level expectations, who makes us want to cuddle up with six-hour reruns of *Pride and Prejudice* until (I am told) we know every intimate crease in Colin Firth's pond-wetted shirt. It was all very simple: *my* Austen was narrowly occupied with matters of the heart (and possibly a man's paycheck), but certainly not health.

And yet, I couldn't ignore the facts. "Health" is mentioned with inescapable frequency in Jane's classic novels, popping up more than a hundred times in those six slim books. From *Northanger Abbey* to *Persuasion*, it's the *other* universally acknowledged truth of Austen's observant pen: "Where health is at stake, nothing else should be considered." The idea is more ubiquitous than marriage proposals, rich gents looking for pretty wives, or bad boys with surnames starting with W. In Austenworld, gaining "health and happiness" in life is just as prized as a one-way ticket to Pemberley. It's one of the recurring themes of *Emma* and the focal point of Austen's last, unfinished novel, *Sanditon* (set—where else?—in a seaside health resort). In Jane's own words, a "picture of health" is painted over the entire canvas of her work: how to lose it and, more importantly, how to obtain it. It influences the way her characters eat, move, think, and feel, giving them either "fresh life and vigour" (à la Lizzie Bennet) or a flabby existence of "ill-health, and a great deal of indolence" (à la Lady Bertram). And if Austen's healthiest characters share one thing, it is that they are all on a sort of *diet* (in the older sense of the word, from the Greek *diaita*, meaning "way of life"). They all embrace a set of healthy lifestyle routines that unfailingly tend to "promote their happiness" as equally and lastingly as falling in love.

Admittedly, I had forgotten the most basic lessons from high school English Lit 101—that Jane Austen wasn't technically a romance novelist at all; she was a *didactic* novelist, a teacher. And what didactic novelists do, when done well, is absolutely magical. They observe life, and all that makes life better, then pass those lessons on to their readers through inspirational clues subtly woven into their stories. Like the best motivational speakers, the ultimate goal of didactic novelists is to paint such a breathtakingly better picture of life on the page that readers are subconsciously inspired to imitate it in reality. That Austen did this with her achingly accurate picture of love is undeniable. Less well known is her equally enviable "picture of health."

Who among us hasn't been inspired, even subliminally, by the effervescent health of Jane's most beloved characters? Lizzie happily goes on a three-mile frolic to Netherfield, her "fine eyes" sparkling the whole way. Catherine Morland eats whenever she likes, guiltlessly enjoying a "healthy appetite" while still managing to slide into her svelte ball gown, no suck-ins ever required. Marianne Dashwood practically glows with energy—"there was a life, a spirit, an eagerness which could hardly be seen without delight." Even dowdy Anne Elliot gets a full-body reboot in *Persuasion*, naturally growing in "bloom and freshness" the more her story progresses. "She was looking remarkably well." It's the sort of statement one hears so often in Jane's novels that a definite pattern emerges. Living in Austenworld doesn't just get you a cushy marriage proposal; it gets you a body guaranteed to turn more than just one top hat.

The inspiration (envy, rather) was unbearable. I had to test this out for myself (seeing that I was on the verge of looking as frumpy as Anne Elliot, circa chapter 1). Piecing together the lifestyle clues in Jane's novels and personal letters, I put myself on the same "diet" of ideas that Austen prescribed for her smartest characters. The way I ate, exercised, and thought about my body, even the way I woke up in the morning and went to bed at night, would be filtered through Austen's unique insights. In short, I would attempt to live within Jane's total "picture of health" this side of the twenty-first century.

I like to think this wasn't as mentally unhinged as traipsing off to Camp Netherfield for Austen-obsessed nutters (though some members of my family would gladly disabuse me of that conviction). My life, after all, is about as far removed from the realities of Regency England as physically possible. Living in a mostly asphalted suburb of South Florida is hardly conducive to frolicking over green pastures with Lizzie Bennet. Furthermore, my other tether to sanity was that I had no intention of stooping to Regency Reenactment Eating—i.e., eating anything other than what I could easily find at my modern American, fluorescently-lit supermarket. Austen's occasional "relish" over a slice of old-English "brawn" (essentially pickled pig's brain) would, alas, be a dieting pleasure I would pass. Thus I assured myself: if Jane's health advice was any less universal, timeless, and truthful as her love advice, I was going to quickly find out. I braced myself for disappointment and disillusion. Instead, I fell "rapidly and deeply in love."

Jane's lifestyle "diet" wasn't just *doable* in the twenty-first century, it was an effortless delight. Whether it was learning how to eat like Emma or exercise like Elizabeth, Austen's health strategies were richer in real-world sense and simplicity than all the health books on my night-stand that year. What's more, Jane seemed to be taking the smartest advice from those books and whittling them down in a way I could easily remember (thanks, in large part, to them being woven into stories I already love, and not just a jumble of boring facts to digest). Getting healthy with Jane truly felt as elegant and graceful as everything else in Austenworld. No starvation tactics, no body sham-ing, no sweaty workouts here, just a calm and civilized strategy for what I naturally needed to return to "a bloom of full health," Regency style.

The Jane Austen Diet is the blueprint for embracing that strategy for yourself—a focus on Jane's little-known food-and-fitness secrets and why they still hold spectacular relevance today. Because while a lot has changed in the last three centuries since Austen lived and wrote (i.e., a "luv-u" text seems more likely than a quilled letter from Captain Wentworth these days), our bodies have certainly not. If anything, what Jane understood about our bodies is more useful, refreshing, and scientifically sensible now than ever before. Austen had the blissful luxury of living before the rise of the modern fad diet. There were no carb revolutions to march in, no zones to fall out of, no calories to count or Paleolithic cavemen to copy. Jane simply approached health, food, and exercise, in the wonderful words of *Persuasion*, "unshackled and free"—free to rely on nature, organic experience, and clever observation to figure out something seemingly impossible, the modern, biological equivalent of marrying Mr. Darcy: how to slim down and eat smart without losing your sanity or self-esteem.

How cleverly Jane figured it all out will be explored in the following pages—a breakfast-to-supper, morning-to-night guide to her Regency recipe to total wellness for the twenty-first century—no bonnets, curtsies, or pickled pig brains required. I promise. More accurately, Jane promises. Her name is mentioned first on this book's cover because these unique and wonderful insights are hers and hers alone. I was simply lucky enough to stumble upon them. Like Mr. Knightly, "I do not pretend to [her] genius." Though if you're looking for a Regency-style boot camp within these covers, for Austen to blow her whistle and whip you back into shape with a loud "drop and give me twenty, dear," I'm afraid you've come to the wrong English spinster. The Austen of incandescent "health and happiness" is the same Austen we've always cherished— the kind, safe, witty brightener of life, always "impatient to restore everybody . . . to tolerable comfort." You've already let her into your heart; it's time to let Jane have a crack at your health. After all, as she most reassuringly pledged: "You will soon be better now . . . You know I always cure you when I come."

"I Can Be No Judge of What the Habit of Self-Doctoring May Do"

Both Jane and I can make a few professional boasts. She, a famous observer of everything that makes humans tick. I, a classically trained chef with a studious soft spot for English literature and food history. Neither of us, however, is a doctor. And while the insights in this book present the timeless body truths in Jane's fiction, passed down to an audience as wide and varied as Austen's modern fans, be sure to consult your trusted apothecary (ahem, physician) if medical questions arise.

"Till this moment, I never knew myself."

—*Pride and Prejudice*

1

UNIVERSAL TRUTHS: BACK TO AUSTEN'S BODY BASICS

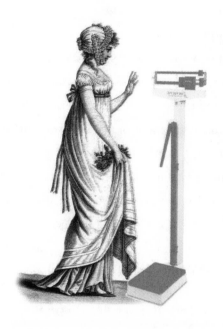

So you want the perfect Jane Austen body? Preferably one of those "happiest of creatures" with Lizzie's sparkling energy, Emma's smart appetite, Elinor's elegant figure, and Marianne's "uncommonly brilliant" skin? Join the club. Getting your own "lovely, blooming, healthful" body straight out of an Austen novel is one of the biggest fantasies in English fiction (on par with meeting your own real-life Mr. Darcy and kindly expecting him to propose twice). And it will remain just another fantasy unless we unlock some of Jane's most important facts first.

I've come to recognize them as Jane's *universal truths*—the Regency body basics repeated throughout her novels, as true today as they were in 1800. They're what the healthiest bodies in Austenworld intuitively understand about health itself. They also happen to clash with some of the peskiest prides and prejudices of the twenty-first century: those "false ideas" about our bodies, as unhelpful to Jane's embrace of life as they've become for us. Because what most of us *believe* healthy bodies should look, act, and think like are simply not Austen's "ideas of happiness" at all. Rather, to obtain both "health and happiness" in Austenworld (and our own) is to allow Jane to set a few things straight. Let's get back to the forgotten body mantras that Lizzie, Darcy, and all the assorted Dashwoods fundamentally "acknowledge to be true":

Universal Truth #1—"Every Body Differed"

First, to line up all the "beautiful" bodies in Austenworld is to clarify one thing: there is no one, perfect Jane Austen body. Healthy, happy, handsome bodies come in "every possible variation of form," says Elinor in *Sense and Sensibility*—a statement anyone who has personally struggled with body-image issues could almost kiss Austen for making. It's such a refreshing alternative to the narrow definitions of *fit* bodies blasted to us in modern magazines, movies, billboards, and the internet. Indeed, to read Austen is to get a much-needed reality check from all that "errant nonsense." One body size does not fit all.

Austen believed it so fully, her novels contain some of the most realistically diverse bodies in English literature. Her leading ladies run the gamut of "attractive" shapes and sizes. There's Anne Elliot on the smaller end of the spectrum with a naturally "slender form" in *Persuasion*, yet Lydia Bennet is equally alluring in *Pride and Prejudice*, being a curvy, "stout, well-grown girl." Harriet Smith joins the body diversity in *Emma*—"She was a very pretty girl . . . short, plump, and fair." So too does Mrs. Croft in *Persuasion*, having a certain "squareness" to her figure, though remaining one of the fittest women in Austenworld nonetheless: full of energy and "blessed with excellent health." Austen herself was naturally "tall and slender" (shaped like a fire poker, some said[1]), but she never forced any of her characters into an identical standard of slimness. Neither does she praise the same "beautiful" body type twice.

These are extraordinary insights for a woman who knew nothing about genetics or DNA. But as science continues to prove, and as Austen hinted three centuries ago, everybody has a "true size for rational happiness"—a biological build as unique as our eye or skin color. My baseline body type is different from yours. Lizzie's is different from Lydia's. Slimming down to your "true size" is certainly welcomed in Austenworld, but one-size-fits-all "standards of perfection" are not. Instead, getting to a "nice comfortable size," being comfortable in your own skin, is Jane's truer message—one repeatedly echoed in *Pride and Prejudice*. When Mr. Darcy snubs Lizzie at the opening ball, finding her body "tolerable, but not hand-some enough to tempt me" ("he had detected with a crit-ical eye more than one failure of perfect symmetry in her form"), Lizzie responds in a way we all universally admire. She doesn't cry in front of a self-loathing mirror or starve herself for a month. She merely laughs it off "among her friends," finding Darcy's narrow beauty standards abso-lutely "ridiculous."

To laugh with Lizzie is to take a step toward sanity, something dearly needed in our own world of critical eyes and impossible "standards of perfection." The fake Photo-shopped bodies in magazines, the digitally tweaked phy-siques in movies, they're all like the ideal "accomplished" woman Miss Bingley blathers on about at Netherfield. "I never saw such a woman," Lizzie rightly rebuffs. She didn't exist in 1813. She doesn't exist today. "Pictures of perfec-tion . . . make me sick and wicked," Austen famously fumed, inviting us all into the exquisite freedom of feeling the same.

Regency Reality Check

If you're having trouble laughing along with Lizzie, researchers at the University of South Florida–Tampa recommend recalibrating your body-perfection standards. Put down the magazine, go to a public place (a shopping mall will suffice, in absence of a Regency ballroom), and do a little people watching.[2] You'll quickly see a wide range of body types and physical beauty that contradict those modern "standards of perfection."

Universal Truth #2—"Wretchedly Thin"

If you think Austen just impolitely spat in the face of every magazine cover model in the country, wait for the next shocker. According to Jane, "thin" bodies aren't automatically "healthy" bodies. In fact—brace yourself—*nobody* is excessively thin and attractive in Austenworld. Take a peek for yourself:

- In *Sense and Sensibility*, as Marianne grows "quite thin," she also "looks very unwell." The same book describes Mrs. Ferrars as a "thin woman . . . without beauty."
- In *Pride and Prejudice*, Miss de Bourgh is repeatedly called "thin" and "sickly." "Who would have thought she could be so thin and small . . . She looks sickly and cross."
- In *Emma*, Miss Bates fears that the once beautiful Jane Fairfax has "grown thin" and is thus "looking very poorly."
- In *Persuasion*, a lovesick "Anne Elliot had been a very pretty girl, but her bloom had vanished early . . . she was [now] faded and thin."

There are more examples, but you're probably growing either confused or uncomfortable—only proof of how deep-rooted our fashionable "thinner is always better" mentality has become. And we're not the only ones. Jane's novels were just as uncomfortably countercultural to the "fashionable world" of Regency England. The early 1800s was one of the first historic periods to embrace a thinness standard as merciless as our own. Both men and women of the era were obsessed with the "tubercular look"—with forcing their bodies into an unnatural state of thinness that could only be achieved through starvation or sickness: to literally look as if they had tuberculosis.[3] Even Marianne gets caught up in the craze in *Sense and Sensibility*: "Confess, Marianne," says Elinor, "is not there something interesting to you in the flushed cheek, hollow eye, and quick pulse of a fever?"—certainly an eerie foreshadowing of the hollow eyes and sickly figures strutting across our fashion runways today.

Austen clearly comprehended how dangerous these ideas are. As she points out in *Northanger Abbey*, there *is* such a thing as being "wretchedly thin"—a biological state as harmful to our health as to our happiness. We can just as easily be "screwed out of health"—yep, Jane said "screwed"—by too little fat on our bodies as by too much. Our brains need a healthy amount of fat to keep us cognitively alive. The same goes for every hard-working cell in our bodies. It's why Austen constantly stresses body "moderation" in her novels, and why a healthier and more beautiful Jane Fairfax is delightfully described in *Emma* as "a most becoming medium, between fat and thin." Emma instinctively knows that this natural-shaped femininity makes Jane Fairfax a serious romantic rival in the novel— an observation still perfectly accurate today. A large 2012 poll conducted by Britain's *Grazia* magazine found that modern men still heartily agree with their Austen male counterparts, preferring the natural beauty of naturally shaped women over the skin-and-bone slightness of size zeros.[4] Lizzie understands it so well, the thought of Darcy (the viscerally hated version) having to marry and kiss the sunken cheeks of Miss de Bourgh fills her with girlish glee. "She looks sickly" and "so thin," says Lizzie, stifling a laugh. "Yes, she will do for him very well." Regency giggle revenge.

A Changing Heroine

Even the film versions of *Pride and Prejudice* reflect how rapidly (and irrationally) our modern body ideals are shrinking. In 1995, BBC's miniseries featured a beautiful and naturally curvy Jennifer Ehle in the role of Elizabeth Bennet. Ten years later, Elizabeth was dramatically sized down into the ultrathin, runway physique of actress Keira Knightley. Deciding which version Austen would have preferred, *"I leave it to my readers' sagacity to determine."*

Universal Truth #3—
"The Whole of the Matter"

If you haven't already noticed, health isn't a narrow matter of weight in Austenworld. Not that weight didn't matter to Jane (her novels certainly contain their fair share of corpulent characters who could afford to lose a few pounds—ahem, Mr. Hurst, Dr. Grant, Mrs. Musgrove). But it wasn't the end-all indicator of health that it's become for us, reflected in the fact that whenever I told my more historically minded friends that I was writing a Jane Austen "diet" book, I would usually brace for the requisite snicker: *but Austen didn't even have a bathroom scale!* Touché. Austen was denied the modern "luxury" of stepping onto a scale to get a daily reminder of how heavy she was, to the accuracy of an ounce. But that, incidentally, made all the difference.

It freed Austen to see something our health-by-numbers culture has practically forgotten—health isn't anything we need a scale to reveal; it's something our bodies manifest naturally, if only we pay attention. Austen explains it best in *Emma*, when Mrs. Weston can't help but notice "how well [Emma] looked last night." "There is health," she says, evident in almost every physical feature. Emma's eyes are clear and "brilliant," her skin radiates with "full health," her figure is "firm" (read: fit) and her "size" is undeniably "pretty."

Mrs. Weston is rephrasing the mainstream medical idea of the Regency era (though one still as relevant today) that health is far more holistic than a number between our toes or a range on a BMI chart. It encompasses the way you look (manifested in Emma's radiant "face and figure") and also the way you feel (equally evident in Emma's "lively" energy and "happy disposition"). Mrs. Weston calls it the whole, "complete" "picture of health"—always far more important to Austen than focusing on any one isolated factor. Let's not forget that Jane knew her English far better than we do: *health* literally means "whole," from the Old English *hale*.

If you've ever wondered why Austen characters so frequently keep tabs on people's physical and emotional "looks," this is why: they are excellent clues for determining whether they are either "in health" or drifting dangerously "out of health"—a lesson we can certainly benefit from today. Fewer guilt trips to our bathroom scales compels us to pay closer attention to our own more realistic and bigger "picture of health"—how our clothes fit, how our skin looks, how our bodies and minds feel. Considered as a whole, and not just a number, it remains the most reliable measure of health in both Austenworld and our own.

"I Will Tell You the Whole Story"

Look at the *whole* story of your health through Austen's holistic eyes. Hop off the scale and start noticing the various body clues Jane recognized as being part of the "bloom of full health"

Skin. Improving "in health" in Austenworld always entails noticing that "your complexion is so improved" too. Jane usually identifies this as a natural "glow" and enhanced "plumpness" to the skin. Which is why *gaining* a little weight is oftentimes a good thing in Jane's novels. In *Northanger Abbey*, Catherine grows more beautiful, "her complexion improved," when "her features were softened by plumpness and colour."

Size. Austen's healthiest heroines never fluctuate dramatically in their weight, preferring to remain at their slimmest "size for rational happiness." Going much beyond this genetic sweet spot, growing either "too thin" or too "heavy-looking" for your individual body type, is an indicator of being "out of health."

Appetite. Are you enjoying a "healthy appetite"? Having a guiltless and rational relationship with food is a crucial component of being in a good "state of health." Jane's smartest characters never starve themselves in order to slim down. Those who do inadvertently damage their bodies and wreck their natural "bloom."

Energy. No character in Austenworld enjoys health without also enjoying "great energy." Feeling a daily surge of "life and vigour," reveling in the "felicity" of a brisk walk or a "lively" dance are some of Jane's most important indicators of overall health. Inversely, chronic "weariness" and a "weakened frame" point just as strongly to "ill health."

Spirits. As health increases so too should your mood. "Good health" and "happy spirits" are intimately linked for Jane, part of her deeper understanding of the mind-body connection (see chapter 7). When happiness is absent, something important has been left out of Austen's "whole story" of health, no matter what the scale says.

That Jane chose to espouse this "whole" picture of health is even more fascinating considering that she *could* have stepped onto a scale if she really wanted to. There was indeed a certain vogue for weighing oneself in the Regency era,[5] though the process was a wee bit humiliating. It involved waddling down to the nearest London warehouse and hopping onto a massive hanging scale: the type usually reserved for weighing heavy wine barrels (because who doesn't like to be the butt of a few body-barrel jokes?). Slightly upping the embarrassment was the fact that a group of goggling onlookers were often standing by, snickering and waiting for the loud announcement of your weight. Needless to say, for most people, this was a novelty, a gag, a one-off experience reserved strictly for the curious and courageous—one of those moments when you could have bought an "I Survived Weighing Myself

Like a Barrel" T-shirt in the gift shop. For others, however, it became a dark spiral for focusing on health as a "number" at the cost of everything else.

The Regency poet and playboy Lord Byron was one of the first victims of this dark side of scales. In 1806, he stepped onto a hanging scale at a wine merchant's shop in London and discovered he was exactly 194 pounds. Deeply humiliated, he became hyper-obsessed with lowering that number, putting himself on an endless round of dangerous starvation diets until he lost over seventy pounds (confirmed again by another compulsive trip to the hanging scale). He continued this damaging cycle of yo-yo dieting until his early death at thirty-six years old—a consequence, many historians now believe, due to abusing his body by obsessively focusing on weight. Byron eventually suspected the same. Over-dieting, he finally realized, was the "cause of more than half our maladies."[6] Obviously, the poor guy wasn't reading Jane Austen.

Universal Truth #4—"Strong Already"

Trusting your body to communicate your "state of health"—trusting your body at all, for that matter—isn't exactly an on-trend topic these days. And small wonder. The modern message couldn't be more aggressively conflicting: our bodies are the real problem, the roadblocks to perfect health. Even the words we use on dieting regimens are a veritable chorus of war cries. We must *battle* the bulge, *fight* cravings, *resist* temptations, *whip* ourselves back into shape. Getting healthy would be easy, yes, if only our wonky carcasses would raise the white flag. Yet Austen, with characteristic elegance, saw things very differently.

Hers is the elegance of the classical approach to health, a body philosophy dating back to ancient Greece and still very much alive in Regency England. An old, intuitive, encouraging idea, it goes something like this: our bodies are naturally strong and resilient. They *want* to be healthy. They are a bit like plants, knowing exactly how to grow without us hovering obsessively over them. Though all plants, of course, need the right environment to flourish. That's where we come in. Our job is to do a little lifestyle gardening, providing the right food and environment for our bodies to do what they do best. Then we step back and stop worrying. Nature has it covered.[7]

Regency doctors called it the *vis medicatrix naturae*, "the healing power of nature," something modern science is just beginning to understand. There are, for instance, stronger antioxidants naturally produced in our bodies (particularly the liver) that rival anything, any superfruit, we could ever consume.[8] Our brains, moreover, are walking pharmacies, naturally dispensing chemicals so potent, they could put many drug companies out of business. Our DNA is programmed for health. We simply need to cooperate.

As Austen affirms in *Mansfield Park*, we are "gifted by nature with strength," which is why you won't find much body bashing in her novels. To attack the thing that makes health attainable didn't make much sense to her. On the contrary, only Austen's nonsensical, comical, and unhealthy characters ever become "over-anxious" about their bodies. Mary Musgrove in *Persuasion*, for example, constantly "suffers" from an "imaginary agitation" of bodily weakness. Even crowded carriage rides "sunk her completely," laying her up on the sofa for most of the day to recover. Mr. Woodhouse in *Emma* labors under a similarly bad body philosophy. For him, people are weak, "delicate plants," needing constant care and obsessive coddling—a self-fulfilling placebo that makes him, in turn, frail and "delicate in [his] own health."

Emma desperately tries to "keep [Mr. Woodhouse] from such thoughts" throughout the novel, as does Austen in almost everything she wrote. From *Pride and Prejudice* to *Persuasion*, her heroines never over-scrutinize their bodies because they rely on one empowering fundamental: that health, for most people, is one of the natural "blessings of existence," the seeds of which they already possess. To approach health like an Austen heroine, therefore, is to look *outside* one's body—at the "habits of life," as Jane puts it, that either weaken or improve what's naturally there to begin with. Everyone in the Regency era had his or her own ideas about what particular "style of living" made health flourish or flounder, as did Austen (her unique insights occupying the following chapters). But the premise remains the same: arrange these external factors correctly and your body, like a resilient plant receiving some much-needed TLC, will naturally reboot toward its healthiest self and size. Your only responsibility along the way, as Lizzie brilliantly observes, is to gently nourish "what is strong already."

Dandelion Detox

Jump-start the healing power of nature with an Austen-approved detox—dandelion tea. Widely available at most supermarkets, dandelion tea was "approved . . . highly" by Jane's family doctor—remarkably, for the same reason it's still prescribed today. It's for "Liver Disorder," says Jane, with modern studies confirming that drinking an occasional cup of dandelion tea can dramatically increase the detoxifying and cleansing power of your liver.[9]

Universal Truth #5—"Mutual Civility"

Truly embracing Austen's *universal truths* for yourself might take some time. Unlearning some of the worst dieting flaws and foibles I picked up from modern life took me time too. Though as far as Jane is concerned, we're in "better company" than we realize. Every character in Austenworld arrives in their stories with their own little flaws and foibles to work through as well (it isn't called _Pride_ and _Prejudice_ for nothing!). But notice that it's only Jane's heroines and heroes who make any effort to improve themselves along the way. The same can't be said for Wickham, Willoughby, or the stubbornly stagnant Mrs. Norris. Instead, the mark of a truly grounded Austenite is simply their willingness to grow, to become a better, stronger, happier version of who they already are. It's the same for Jane's approach to health.

Not every Austen beauty bursts onto the page with "fresh life and vigour" like Lizzie Bennet. Anne Elliot, for one, requires a few chapters to go from frumpy and "faded" to gradually "having the bloom and freshness of youth restored." Marianne Dashwood likewise has some bad body beliefs to unlearn too, mostly regarding the pitfalls of starvation diets. But sooner or later, "improvement of health" is *always* part of Austen's package for a happily ever after.

To borrow Lizzie's endearing language, your body naturally "improves upon acquaintance." The more you know how it works and what it needs to thrive, the better this cooperative relationship of health becomes. As it was with Darcy, "from knowing [it] better, [its] disposition was better understood." You don't have to love your body right from the start—love at first sight? Don't make Lizzie laugh! But you do have to respect it—respect it enough to deem it worthy of wonderful improvements. Just a small, polite bow of "mutual civility." Just the beginning of every great Austen romance.

"We agreed that the best thing we could
do is begin eating . . . and instantly
began our Devouring Plan . . . ."
—*Juvenilia*

2

"OUR DEVOURING PLAN": A HEROINE'S GUIDE TO FOOD

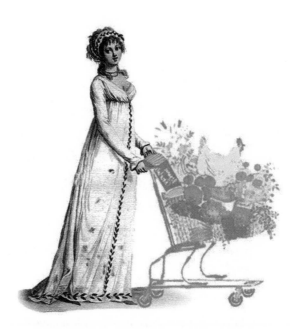

You can begin by unlacing your mental corset. Food is one of the few things in Austenworld not governed by a "strict rule of right." Jane advises no prim-and-proper parallels to our modern food regulations, no Regency equivalents to the calories, zones, points, charts, nutrition labels, and glycemic indexes that keep our dietary posture in check.

For a gal who knows more about life's convoluted "rules of conduct" (from how low to curtsy to how to successfully flirt with a hand fan), when it comes to food—just one of the foundations of life itself—Jane seems as relaxed as a Regency rogue. "I'm sure I do not care," says Catherine Morland in *Northanger Abbey*, "It is all the same to me what I eat."

Eek. Such shocking indifference! We'd half expect it to engender a world full of flabby flubdubs, lazy eaters with all manner of horrendous dining habits. What Jane gives us instead is the real shocker. Hers is a world where loosened attitudes toward food aren't the undoing of healthy heroines, they are the making of them: where the less one says and stresses over food, the more it effortlessly "rested in its proper place," where "rational creatures" are free to enjoy a "healthy appetite" without ever being controlled by it. The result is one of literature's least complicated and most enviable approaches to food on record—one of the rare moments when you can realistically imagine Jane Austen doing a sofa-slouched impersonation of Scarlett O'Hara: "Food? Oh, fiddle-dee-dee! Mustn't fuss about *that*, silly."

Easy for her to say. No doubt we'd all obtain the same nirvanic attitude toward food if *we* lived in the rosy glow of the Regency era. One can only imagine the extent of our difficult food choices: *Dear me. Shall I go strawberry picking with Emma or nut gleaning amongst the hedgerows with Louisa Musgrove?* Romance novel reality check.

What can outdated Aunt Jane and her frilly tea cakes possibly know about our modern struggles with food?

Actually, not seeing those cakes for their calories is precisely what makes Jane's food philosophies so exquisitely valuable to us today. Food was never a caloric number for Austen, a soulless fragment of carbon energy to count and quickly scarf down. It was one of the dynamic "comforts of life," and therefore something to develop a lifelong, rational relationship with. Relationships are all that really matter to Jane anyway. And it's not exactly a Pulitzer Prize–winning statement to say that she was rather good at describing them. Austen's best romances have a Zen-like balance between comfort and control (i.e., Elinor falling head over heels in love with Edward while staunchly remaining "mistress of myself"). The same is true for Jane's approach to food. Love isn't the only desire capable of going astray in Austenworld. Bad food romances are just as common. For all her misguided Lydia Bennets, characters who live only to flirt, there are just as many Mr. Hursts, tubby bon vivants who "lived only to eat." So it's no coincidence that Austen's heroines, the characters who love the wholest, also eat the healthiest, enjoying the edible "pleasures of life" without allowing them to interrupt life itself.

How they do it, blithely bouncing from one Regency meal to the next, at first seems lost in the airy mystique of Austen's imagination (somewhat like Lizzie's elusive formula for falling in love *and* getting fabulously rich). Jane, however, is a bit more pragmatic when it comes to eating like a heroine. It's scattered throughout most everything she wrote, an elegant diet of mind-sets, ideas, and mental tactics. She calls it "our Devouring Plan" in one of her earliest stories, recognizing even as a child that every heroine needs a thoughtful strategy for tackling food with "tolerable composure."[1] Later in her novels, "our Devouring Plan" would become Austen's own safety net for always keeping one's relationship with food in its "proper place." To unlock its secrets is to strike at the heart of healthy eating, no matter the century. Time to throw out your calorie corset and rewire the way you approach food. Time to eat like it's 1811!

1. "Tolerably Detached"

For starters, let's clarify what I mean by developing a Regency *relationship* with food (lest I be hanged, drawn, and quartered by the Jane Austen Society for willful ineptitude). Because as every Austen scholar knows, Jane never gets gushy over food. If anything, she constantly keeps her heroines from ever developing what she would call a "warm attachment" to it—a fact emotional eaters have never quite forgiven her for. The only truly healthy food relationships in Austenworld are the ones, in effect, that keep food at an emotional arm's length. Lizzie even refuses to talk about it too much (rather disappointing Mr. Hurst in the process, a man obviously looking forward to spending the evening discussing the giddy delights of French "ragout" with her). It's the same in *Sense and Sensibility*.

Try as she might, Mrs. Jennings can't make picky foodies out of Elinor and Marianne—she was "only disturbed that she could not make them choose their own dinners at the inn, nor extort a confession of their preferring salmon to cod, or boiled fowls to veal cutlets."

We want to shout, "Get a grip, girls—it's only food!" But that's exactly Jane's point. Food is meant to be regarded with minimalistic mental energy in Austenworld, "with a proper air of indifference." If there are to be any complicated fantasies, warm, fuzzy feelings, or periodic swoonings, they are reserved for Mr. Pemberton Plumptre, your handsome neighbor down the lane, not the plum pudding in your larder. Jane brilliantly understood the psychological pitfalls of doing so—to get any more personal, intimate, and emotional with food is to inevitably fall into dieting dangers.

Traci Mann explains it with perfect modern parallels in *Secrets from the Eating Lab*.[2] Specifically, most people tend to be terrible at resisting daily food temptations when their relationship to food gets too touchy-feely. Imagine a box of doughnuts passed around the office, Mann tells us. To regard them with simple, Austen-style indifference (they're *just* breakfast items, round pastries in a cardboard container) is to dramatically lessen their power. On the other hand, to overthink them, to remember your past doughnut romance—how the frosting melted in your mouth, how buttery-scrumptious it all smelled, how the first sugary bite made you feel—is to back yourself into a complicated corner of cravings nearly impossible to resist. You'll end up eating the doughnut (likely plural) every time. It's why Austen constantly reminds us to keep our emotions away from food. Keep "everything as natural and simple as possible," insists Mrs. Elton in *Emma*.

If only Dr. Grant got the memo. The corpulent clergyman of *Mansfield Park* is one of the worst food romancers in Austenworld. He obsesses over food and prioritizes it with comical exuberance. "The business of his own life is to dine," to "eat, drink, and grow fat." Those familiar with the novel know what follows. Thanks to a repeated "habit of self-indulgence," constant stressing and "quarrelling" over food and "three great institutionary dinners in one week," he eventually succumbs to "apoplexy and death." Though as much as we may giggle at Dr. Grant's demise (hard not to when Austen practically calls him a balloon "that would soon pop off"), chances are we've all gone a bit Grant-like bonkers over food too.

Just think back to the last time you went to the grocery store hungry, or the last restrictive diet you struggled to maintain, or even the last time you skipped lunch and drove past a billboard advertising a double-decker burger and large fry. How good were you at achieving a "proper air of indifference" toward food? Spectacularly terrible, no doubt. Fact is, most of us are absolute nutters when we're hungry, ravenously unable to concentrate on anything besides a running internal monologue of Food-Food-Food-No-I-Couldn't-Possibly-Oh-Look-More-Food.

It's something science has known for decades, that the more we restrict food in our lives and diets, the more we're doomed to obsess over it. Blame it on biology and your body's keen knack at keeping you alive, but there are few things more hopeless at fighting than the complex chemistry of your natural hunger hormones.[3] Healthy food detachments are only possible, paradoxically, when you're eating enough.

That Jane grasped this biological truth is evident by how often she reminds her characters to eat, to eat in a way that is fully, naturally satisfying. Catherine Morland's embrace of life, her sprightly vigor, is regularly fueled by "a good appetite." She eats when she's hungry, even late at night after a ball. It's the same appetite respect Emma Woodhouse is expected to have. One of the conditions for her going to the Coles' evening party was her solemn promise that if she came home "hungry . . . she would take something to eat." Emma passes on the same wisdom to a hangry Frank Churchill, knowing that "eating" was "often the cure of such incidental complaints." "Go eat," she tells him, "another slice of cold meat, another draught of Madeira and water, will make you nearly on a par with the rest of us." To get yourself likewise "on par" with Austen's heroines is to admit that you're not a dieting automaton with no biological needs. It's okay, and even advisable, to begin your relationship with food where Jane begins chapter 9 of *Mansfield Park*—with one honest and refreshing acknowledgement: "It was first necessary to eat."

I Am Woman, See Me Eat

Readers today tend to forget how progressive Jane's eating encouragements were for the time. Regency "fashions" promoted exactly the opposite, labeling eating itself as somehow an indelicate, unwomanly thing to do. "A woman should never be seen eating or drinking," said Lord Byron in 1812, insisting that if she *must* eat (what a thought!) it should be something inherently "feminine and becoming."[4] Try finding *that* label in the supermarket. It was one of the first cultural fads that Jane ridiculed with biting wit in *Love and Friendship*, a short story written in her teens. "Never, never . . . will I so demean myself," says one of its stupider characters, with "the mean and indelicate employment of eating and drinking." That Jane laughed at this idea so early on only proves how accurately she understood her main subject— love. A realistic love life, in fact, demands a realistic relationship with food. Scientists first discovered the connection in the 1940s, in one of the first experiments into calorie restriction. They found that the more people "dieted" (eating only minimal amounts of food), the less romantically inclined they felt. Though the test subjects were all young and healthy, the joys of falling in love became "too much trouble" when they weren't getting enough to eat. Instead, food became their new passion, the only thing they could think, talk, and obsess over.[5] That Jane's heroines *don't* do this, that they spend more time thinking about love and not about food, is actually the best evidence that they aren't dieting in the traditional sense. Because whatever people "might think," Jane told her sister in 1813, "an empty Stomach" is not "the most favourable for Love."

2. "Harmonized By Distance"

If distance makes the heart grow fonder in Austenworld, it also makes for much healthier eating habits. That is, there's a reason why food is only brought out during specific mealtimes in Jane's novels, and almost exclusively enjoyed in the boundaries of the "dining-parlour." The image of Lizzie slumping into the kitchen and snatching a pork-pie snack is such an un-Austen thought, Mrs. Bennet is positively rankled by the idea—"she assured him with some asperity that . . . her daughters had nothing to do in the kitchen." The idea was pervasive during the Regency era. It wasn't deemed proper, polite, or civilized for gentlefolk to be constantly surrounded by the sights, smells, or sounds of food. Regency kitchens were thus placed as far away as physically possible from everyday living quarters. One real-life Pemberley estate, Kedleston Hall in Derbyshire, even managed to distance its kitchen over sixty-five yards from its dining room, more than half the size of a football field.[6] And while honesty forbids categorizing this as anything but pure Regency snobbery (footmen don't get paid for nothing, silly!), it must be said that setting up all these physical barriers to food practically eliminated mindless eating. Who can brainlessly binge when a trip to the pantry involves a mini-triathlon?

The modern contrasts, of course, are striking. "Open concept" home designs have practically plopped kitchens into our living rooms, with everyone's refrigerator now an effortless sock-slide away. Today, to find yourself on the wrong end of a ravishing ice cream craving is to open the freezer with one pinky finger (Jane, comparatively, first had to stroll down to the dairy and find herself an obliging cow). Needless to say, all this modern "convenience" has made for a world where food is more accessible, more thoughtlessly tempting than ever: where we can all too easily stare into those empty cartons of Rocky Road Double-Fudge Remorse and wonder how they got into our laps in the first place. Let's face it, we all desperately need a bit of Regency-style distance between us and our food. And as science is observing, we don't need a Kedleston Hall (or a cow) to do it.

Researchers at the University of Illinois have discovered that even small distances and tiny obstacles tend to be incredibly effective at halting mindless snacking. In a study involving a container of chocolate candy (and how far people had to reach to get it), participants found themselves munching far more frequently when the container was placed at an easy arm's reach than when the same container was moved mere feet away. Unbelievably, the physical drag of getting up and walking a few steps was enough of an obstacle to drastically minimize thoughtless eating.[7]

It all comes down to, as Austen would say, "a great deal of indolence." People naturally don't like to work too hard at procuring food (especially when they're not that hungry in the first place). It's a great reminder for embracing your inner Regency laziness, to become a "rational, though languid" eater naturally unwilling to traverse the curvy corridors of your own Kedleston Hall. Translating that into the twenty-first century starts by limiting the number of convenience foods at home. They make eating a little *too* convenient. And if you find yourself reaching for that carton of ice cream, don't reach for the freezer. Instead, create a Regency-style barrier. Drive (or better yet, walk) down to your local ice cream parlor for a single serving. Then again, you'll probably think twice about the whole expedition, exhaling along with Austen, "I have not the heart for it."

3. "Inseparably Connected"

The Western world now enjoys access to the cheapest, most abundant food on the planet, with one sobering irony—all that inexpensive abundance makes it hard to properly enjoy it. As supermarkets brim with cheap food in bulging bags and plastic packages, it's difficult not to buy into the general illusion, to treat food as cheaply as it costs. Oddly enough, Regency well-to-dos had a very similar problem.

Compared to revolutionary France, food was fantastically abundant in early nineteenth-century England. Cartoons of the era glorified it, depicting rotund English diners devouring mountainous buffets of food, gigantic roast beefs, immoderately large puddings, and fishbowl-sized pints of beer (while their silly French neighbors fought over a single frog to sauté).[8] And no one pigged out on Britain's edible bounty more than the era's eponymous overeater, George IV, the Prince Regent. Usually depicted with satirical, beach ball proportions, George liked his dinners like he liked his mistresses: large and lots of 'em. They were gorging extravaganzas (the dinners, not the mistresses): four-hour marathons of continuous feasting on dozens of main dishes and desserts.[9] It seems to be the fate of all prosperous cultures, regardless of century. To be surrounded by a land of edible plenty is to instinctively begin to overeat. It's only natural. Rather, it's the unnatural consequence of separating ourselves from nature itself, from where our food comes from and the real cost of eating it.

Jane Austen experienced a much closer connection. She grew up on a farm in Hampshire that was practically self-supporting.[10] She knew the immense work involved in coaxing the earth to produce something edible, but she also knew the joys. Her letters are full of the little excitements of kitchen gardening: finding the first apricot in the orchard, turning the last summer berries into jam. Read them carefully and Austen's novels become an enchanting hymn to England's agricultural heritage, particularly expressed in

Emma. Who can forget the "superior" pork raised right on the Hartfield estate, or the "ripening" strawberries and "wholesome" apples that come directly from Mr. Knightley's farm? A farm that inspires one of the rarest narratorial rhapsodies in all of Austen's fiction: "At the bottom of this bank, favourably placed and sheltered, rose the Abbey-Mill Farm, with meadows in front, and the river making a close and handsome curve around it. It was a sweet view—sweet to the eye and the mind. English verdure, English culture, English comfort, seen under a sun bright."

For Jane, to feel "inseparably connected" with food's earthy roots is to naturally ensure a healthy respect for it. Overeating (just for the heck of it) proves difficult when you understand the meaningful struggle behind the meal. And while we can't make the time-leap back to the rolling farmlands of Regency England, we can still return to an Austen-esque appreciation for what we eat. We just need to recalibrate our basic food consciousness by remembering how precious food really is. Try visiting a local farmer's market, planting a vegetable garden, or baking something from scratch. Reacquaint yourself with the real cost of food. You'll soon start respecting (and reducing) what winds up on your fork.

4. "Dining in Company"

For novels with more meal scenes and "famous dinners" than one can shake a fork at, one thing happens with astonishing rarity—an Austen character eating alone. It only happens twice in Jane's novels, both times standing out like glaring anomalies. Willoughby's rushed lunch for one near the end of *Sense and Sensibility*, for example, seems almost profligate. Likewise, Mr. Weston's solitary dinner in *Emma* appears to unsettle the entire village. Note that he must satisfy "inquiries" that his lonely meal wasn't too unbearable. Poor soul. Modern readers tend to ignore these atypical details. They're so drastically different from what we love about Austen's novels: the social meals, the endless dinner invitations, the long tables, the lively conversations amidst all that lovely "eating, drinking, and laughing together."

We love it because most of us have temporarily lost it. Our relationship with food can now, we are told, be only two basic things: food can either be fuel (for those who *eat to live*) or food can be pleasure (for those who *live to eat*). Notice both views will probably leave you eating alone. We don't think it matters, but Austen says it does. Mrs. Bennet brags about dining "with four-and-twenty families" for good reason. It's something other cultures and other countries still understand—that there's a built-in safety valve when we eat "in company." Food becomes more than just fuel, more than just pleasure, when we eat with others. It becomes a binder for the relationships that matter most (especially to Jane)—love, friendship, family, community.

It follows that large quantities of food are never hoarded for solitary binges in Jane's novels; they are always shared amongst friends. When Mrs. Goddard in *Emma*, for instance, receives a sizable present of poultry ("a beautiful goose: the finest goose Mrs. Goddard had ever seen"), she immediately invites "three teachers . . . to sup with her," thereby eliminating the temptation for isolated overeating. This is one of the main reasons for why food is never something to be feared or forbidden in Austen's fiction. It simply isn't necessary. Food becomes less personally "sinful" or "guilt-ridden" the more it is communally divided— hence Jane's fondness for giving dining room occupancy numbers in her novels. It's fourteen in the Bennet's case. That's how many chairs their dinner table can snugly accommodate. The more the merrier (and the mentally healthier). "He did look upon a tolerably large eating-room as one of the necessaries of life."

The further benefits of eating "in company" will be explored in the following chapter. For now, just remember that to eat alone in Austenworld means to exclude something crucial from a meal. There's safety in numbers.

Jane has so much more to say about food, and we'll get into specifics in subsequent chapters. But there's something we need to clarify before we close. According to Austen, there is nothing wrong, nothing unusual or unhealthy about truly enjoying food. That eating can be, and often is, very enjoyable is a fact repeatedly expressed in her personal letters. "I always take care to provide such things as please my own appetite," she unabashedly wrote. Added is her adorably frank comment about apple pies being a "considerable part" of her "domestic happiness." Jane wasn't interested in what she called "self-mortification." Constant denials were, for her, as unhealthy as constant indulgences. "What some call health, if purchased by perpetual anxiety about diet, isn't much better than tedious disease"—a quote often attributed to one of Austen's favorite poets, Alexander Pope. And Jane echoes the sentiment exactly. Behold Mrs. Jennings' delightful mulberry memory in *Sense and Sensibility*—"Delaford is a nice place . . . quite shut in with great garden walls that are covered with the best fruit-trees in the country: and such a mulberry tree in one corner! Lord! how Charlotte and I did stuff the only time we were there!"

Food pleasures should never be a priority, but neither can pleasure be excluded from food, especially since pleasure appears to be a crucial puzzle piece to digesting it properly. First demonstrated in a now classic experiment from the 1970s, when participants in the study were given familiar foods they actually enjoyed, the rate of healthy iron absorption from the meal was 50 percent greater than when they were given foods that were less familiar and less appetizing.[11] Pleasure seems to cue our bodies to metabolically make the best of things, to take full advantage of food's nutritional offerings. But balance has always been key: the yin and yang of stoic dieting *sense* on the one hand and pleasurable *sensibility* on the other, the only way to approach food happily and wholly. People have said the same thing, slightly differently, for generations. Not too long ago in Britain there was a wonderfully common saying that probably expressed it best: "A little of what you fancy does you good."[12] Austen couldn't agree more.

AUSTEN EATS: BREAD

A few things happen with such routine predictability in Jane's novels, you can bet your last copper farthing that somewhere in Austenworld, somebody is quite merrily doing the following: dropping a curtsy, pouring tea, visiting, planning a ball, visiting, dancing with a cad at said ball, begging for a ditty on the pianoforte, generally "astonished" at something or other, visiting, squealing with the certainty that someone will be married by Michaelmas. So it wouldn't hurt to add one more to the well-established list, to "all those little matters on which the daily happiness of private life depends." It's as simple and spontaneous as all the rest: Austen characters eat bread every day without an ounce of dieting hesitation.

"I Hope You Will Eat Some of This Toast"

You already know this, even if you've never picked up one of her novels. Every Austen film adaptation has one: the usual breakfast scene with Regency rich folk gossiping through prim mouthfuls of buttered toast. Hollywood set designers have done their research. Enjoying "a bit of bread" on a daily basis was an expected luxury of living well in Austen's England. So much so, Jane tends to offer bread *more* regularly as her characters develop increasingly elegant lifestyles.

Case in point: When Catherine Morland returns to her humbler home after living the high life at Northanger Abbey, she can hardly stop reminiscing about the delicious bread she regularly ate there, cueing the eye rolls of her less ritzy relations: "I did not quite like, at breakfast, to hear you talk so much about the French bread at Northanger," says her mother. Then there's Fanny Price, who experiences the exact opposite fate. Accustomed to the fresh baked goods served at Mansfield Park, she goes into temporary bread withdrawals when staying with her less privileged family in Portsmouth. She does, however, manage to tide herself over by coaxing her brothers to fetch a daily supply of "biscuits and buns" from the local bakery. There are "little privations" one doesn't suffer through in Austenworld. Going breadless is one of them. Small wonder: to be "without bread to eat" is Jane's byword for total life bombing.

To say we've come far in our attitude toward bread would be the dieting understatement of the century. Bread?—in a *diet* book? Frankly, I could have started this chapter, "Austen Eats: Regency Fish Head Ragout" and gotten far fewer nervous giggles. Bread is something us moderns only indulge in between our diets—brief moments of carb- and gluten-gorging insanity. *Between* is the most realistic word, given the fact that going totally breadless throughout life seems to be the dieting equivalent of trying to hold your breath underwater. Some can go longer than others (yay, them), but most mortals are bound to pop up eventually, usually hyperventilating into the nearest bagel.

Can't eat it healthfully, can't live without it happily is the epitaph we seem doomed to keep etching over our modern bread fates. The idea of incorporating bread into a healthy, guiltless lifestyle seems as foreign and far-off as everything else on Austen's list of "normal" Regency routines. No one bobs a curtsy anymore, and yet Jane's basic bread beliefs are more alive and normal than you might think.

Anyone who has visited France has already seen walking examples of it. The image of elegant Parisians strolling home with fresh baguettes tucked under their armsis iconic for good reason. The French are famous for enjoying, like nineteenth-century Austenites, their daily "bit of bread." And to the eyes of modern Americans, they seem to pull it off with magical impunity. Somehow, their regular intake of croissants doesn't automatically get stuccoed onto their stomachs and, bar the rare medical diagnosis, they've largely managed to avoid being even remotely interested in going gluten free. Healthy French eaters refuse to live without the joys of bread, said Mireille Guiliano in *French Women Don't Get Fat*, certainly one of the more shocking and enviable tenants in the book.[1] What's really going on under the surface, however, is a set of traditional guidelines about eating bread, and eating it correctly, that the French have naturally inherited. Centuries of loving those baguettes have taught the French how to live with them healthfully. Go deeper into Austen's fiction and we find the same thing.

Living at the height of historical bread-eating wisdom, Jane knew there was a real difference between "bad . . . bread" and good, just as there are bad ways and good ways of eating it. To flippantly ban it all, just because we've forgotten how to properly enjoy it, would be seen by Austen as "intolerably stupid." Rather, a simple return to Regency bread basics is all we need to rethink our modern wheat worries and get the proverbial *staff of life* back into our own. Remember, nobody goes entirely breadless while Jane's around: "Could I bear to see her want while I had a bit of bread to give her?" Perish the thought!

"A Slight, Thin Sort of Inclination"

There are, of course, Regency bread faux pas to first consider. For one, this isn't the era to turn up with a party-sized pumpernickel and spinach dip, expecting everybody to tear off massively big bites. *"Good heavens . . . how can you think of such a thing?"* The Regency era might have been full of unabashed bread lovers, but they approached it with more—shall we say?—"scruples of delicacy." Because to elegantly enjoy bread like Austen is, first and foremost, a matter of portion size.

A slice of bread, whether served at Northanger Abbey or Mansfield Park, always meant a *thin* slice. The thinner the better. Visitors to England commented on the custom. "The slices of bread and butter which they give you with your tea are as thin as poppy leaves" noted a German traveler in 1782, adding that, though small, they are "incomparably good."[2]

Bread was truly one of the greatest less-is-more foods on Regency tables. To tear off bigger chunks from the loaf would have "bordered too much on inelegance." Fact is, the Regency poor had no choice but to live on bread alone in order to survive. Richer folk (and those who strived to live like them) could afford to eat it in refined moderation, hence Miss Bates' indirect boast on how small her regular order is at the baker's in *Emma*: "for what is our consumption of bread, you know? Only three of us." Her rhetorical point was it's very little. *Daily enjoyed yet daintily eaten* is the bread balance every conscientious Austenite aims for.

"The Usual Practice of Elegant Females"

It's still considered "posh" and elegantly upper class to eat bread with dainty restraint in modern-day England. There, the proper way of tackling anything bready served with a spread (be it toast with jam, or rolls with butter) involves first breaking off a small, mouth-sized bite of bread with your fingers and spreading butter/jam just on that tiny bit. Only after you've eaten *that* piece can you repeat the process, starting over with another mouth-sized bite to break off, spread, and eat.[3] It all makes for a purposefully slow and very mindful way of eating bread that seriously limits the likelihood of overeating it. The "vulgar" alternative, however, is to slather all the butter/jam over the bread in one go, then chomp your way through the whole slice—no doubt finishing off the slice (and reaching for another) before realizing you've even begun.

Jane knew that most of us only experience a natural craving for "a bit of bread," not an entire bakery full. To use her expression, one can feel "perfectly satisfied" over even small servings of bread. This idea was validated by Paul Rozin, professor of psychology at the University of Pennsylvania, who found that bread portion sizes can be easily manipulated without us ever feeling deprived. In a real-world experiment in 2005, Rozin closely observed the eating habits of residents at one apartment building where, three times a week, a large supply of soft pretzels was put out in the lobby for the residents' enjoyment. On normal days, people reached for a whole pretzel—that is, until Rozin had the pretzels cut in half. Now totally free to take two halves, people automatically cut back, grabbing half a pretzel instead, what they naturally viewed as a single serving.[4]

Applying the same *half rule* to your bread choices will get you closer to a more Regency-appropriate relationship with bread. Whether that's half a bagel instead of a whole, a thin slice instead of a thick one, or three crackers instead of six, bread is one of the few things Austen would totally recommend learning to "love by halves."

Doing "Full Justice" To Bread

What *type* of bread did Austen eat? Better yet, what did she avoid? Because while Jane certainly enjoyed her regular bit of toast, bun, and buttered crumpet, not all bread was created equal in her mind.

The Regency era was one of the first pioneers of adding what we would now call *chemical additives* to bread. A popular craze for whiter, cheaper loaves (sound familiar?) prompted bakers to bulk up their bread with all manner of questionable, and oftentimes dangerous, ingredients. Powdered chalk and alum were the usual adulterants, but lime, ground animal bones, and the occasional dose of white lead were also suspected of being surreptitiously slipped in as well.[5] "The bread I eat in London, is a deleterious paste," complained the novelist Tobias Smollett in 1771, "mixed up with chalk, alum and bone-ashes; insipid to the taste, and destructive to the constitution." The "baker," he added, "is obliged to poison" us all.[6] Austen suspected the same. When visiting London, one was all too liable to "eat very bad baker's bread," she told her sister in 1813.

Her suspicions could just as easily apply today. We might not find the odd "pulverized pelvic bone" listed on its labels, but the modern bread aisle is, in very real ways, an additive blast from the Regency past. Questionable ingredients are now being added to bread with the same historic gusto, with some of the most questionable of all including:

- 🔒 **Gluten**. This is *not* the natural gluten (the organic protein) found in wheat, oats, barley, and rye—and present in humanity's bread since the dawn of eating it. Rather, it means *vital gluten* has been added to the dough: a concentrated, highly processed form of powdered gluten chemically engineered for the mass bread market. Adding such artificially high levels of gluten allows bread companies to create light, springy loaves faster than ever before. It's also suspected of being one of the prime culprits in the modern rise in gluten sensitivity and celiac disease.[7]
- 🔒 **Potassium Bromate**. Often lurking as "bromated flour" on ingredient labels, potassium bromate might help modern bread loaves rise and increase in volume, but it is banned in most of Europe, Canada, and Japan for its links to causing cancer in lab rats.[8]
- 🔒 **Butylated Hydroxyanisole (BHA)**. The jury is still out on the overall safety of BHA—a popular preservative used to increase the shelf life of bread—but the National Institutes of Health now concludes that it is "reasonably anticipated to be a human carcinogen."[9]

Obviously, very little has changed since Austen warned her sister about the likelihood of eating "very bad . . . bread." Which is probably why she so eagerly reminds us of the simple solution. In *Emma*, there are repeated references to a bakery—a good, honest, wholesome bakery—in the village of Highbury. This is where Miss Bates buys her dependable loaves and where "dawdling children" tend to cluster "round the baker's little bow-window eyeing the gingerbread." Austen even gives us the name of the baker's wife (a notably rare moment of giving details below the hierarchy of the upper classes)—the "extremely civil and obliging" Mrs. Wallis, a woman who does "full justice" to her baked goods. What that meant for Austen (doing "full justice" to bread) is what it has always meant: abiding by a traditional way of making bread that hasn't changed since Mrs. Wallis lit her bread ovens three centuries ago. That is, natural ingredients kneaded, leavened, and baked normally. Bread makers in both the Regency era and today have never needed more than four basic ingredients (flour, yeast, water, salt) to create a delicious loaf. Adding much more than that, seeing fifteen or twenty or thirty ingredients on a bread label, and you're likely heading into bad bread territory no matter the century.

"Real, Honest, Old-fashioned" Bread

Despite never uttering the phrase "gluten sensitive" in her life, much of the bread Austen ate was remarkably gluten friendly. Before the availability of fast-acting yeast, Regency bakers routinely leavened their breads by mixing old chunks of unbaked dough into new.[10] Once in, the leftover dough (full of yesterday's yeast) would naturally start rising the new batch, creating the same soft, airy, springy loaves we still love today—with a slight tang from the wild yeast and friendly bacteria. While the process required far more time and patience—anywhere between twelve to sixteen hours to create a fully leavened loaf—it also came with simultaneous health benefits. Wheat bread made in this traditional manner (known as *sourdough* to us) is much easier to digest. Sourdough's long fermentation breaks down the natural gluten in the wheat, creating loaves with dramatically lower amounts of that tricky protein. So much so, a 2007 study found that breads made with this sourdough technique had such reduced gluten levels, they were well under the FDA's legal guidelines for "gluten free" foods.[11] It certainly explains why Austen believed that well-made bread was so easy on the stomach. With her mother suffering from queasiness and a wobbly stomach after a long journey in 1798, Austen happily reported that, nevertheless, "my mother . . . ate some bread several times."

Jane's Grocery List

"We . . . walked about snugly together and shopp'd."
Choose "thin-sliced" options for all bread. Leave the rest
(big, rustic, thick-cut loaves) for those Regency peasants
and their "vulgar relations." *Snooty sniff.*

Watch out for "bad . . . bread" with dubious chemical
additives. Take special care to avoid bread with words
such as "gluten" or "vital gluten," "bromated," or "BHA" on
its ingredient label.

Buy traditionally made sourdough whenever possible.
Ask your bakery if the dough was made using a natural
"starter" with a long fermentation—then apologize for
being "impertinently curious."

Bath Buns

Makes 12

"It was an excellent journey . . . We ate three
of the buns in the course of that stage, the
remaining three made an elegant entertainment
for Mr. and Mrs. Tilson who drank tea with us."
—Austen's letters

Served warm at breakfast or tea, these buns were a favorite treat of Jane's when staying in Bath. One of the most iconic English buns, they're squishy soft with a subtle sweetness from the raisins and milky glaze.

DOUGH:

1 packet (¼ ounce) active dry yeast

2 teaspoons, plus 2 tablespoons sugar, divided

¼ cup warm water

½ cup milk

3 tablespoons unsalted butter, divided

2 cups bread flour (not all-purpose—no cheating!)

Zest of 1 lemon

½ teaspoon salt

1 egg, beaten

⅓ cup raisins

Parchment paper

GLAZE:

2 tablespoons milk

2 tablespoons sugar

Sugar pearls for decorating

1. Put the yeast and 2 teaspoons of sugar in a small bowl. Pour in the warm water and leave until the yeast is bubbly and frothy, about 5 to 10 minutes.

2. Heat the milk and 2 tablespoons butter in the microwave until butter has just melted. Allow to cool slightly.

3. Mix the flour, lemon zest, salt, and 2 tablespoons of sugar in a large bowl. Make a well in the center of the flour, then pour in the warm (not hot) milk and melted butter, the yeasty liquid, and the beaten egg. Mix with a wooden spoon until just combined. Dough will be thick and sticky.

4. Cover the bowl with a damp dishcloth and leave in a warm place for the dough to rise and triple in size, about 1½ hours. (If your house is cold, try this slightly zany—but fail-proof—technique: run your empty clothes dryer for one minute, place the bowl of dough inside, shut the door and giggle at the cleverness of you.)

5. Meanwhile, generously dust a small work surface with flour and get a small handful of raisins at the ready. Line a 9 x 13-inch baking dish with parchment paper.

6. Dust your hands with flour and dump the dough onto the floured surface. Shape the dough into a short log. Cut the log into 4 equal pieces, then cut each piece into 3 smaller pieces (to make 12 pieces of dough in total).

7. Take one piece of dough, pat it slightly flat, and drop a few raisins in the center. Gather the sides of the dough, stretching them up over the raisins. Pinch to seal and flip over to reveal a smooth ball of dough. Place the ball smooth-side up on the baking dish and repeat with the remaining dough, lining them up 3 across and 4 down.

8. Brush the tops of the dough balls with 1 tablespoon of melted butter. Cover the dish with plastic wrap and return to a warm place for the balls to double in size, about 30 minutes. Preheat oven to 400°F.

9. Remove the plastic wrap and bake for 6 to 8 minutes, or until the buns are golden brown. While baking, make the glaze: stir the milk and sugar in a small bowl until combined.

10. Remove the buns from the oven and brush the glaze over their tops twice. While the glaze is still wet, push a few raisins into the top of each bun, making a shallow well in the center for the raisins to nestle in. Sprinkle some pearl sugar over the raisins and serve the buns warm.

"What a delightful place Bath is."
—*Northanger Abbey*

"It would be such a delicious scheme . . .
and completely do for us at once."

—*Pride and Prejudice*

3
THE PEMBERLEY MEAL PLAN

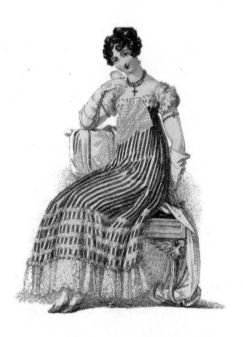

One can almost hear Mr. Collins wheezing nervously in the background . . .

"Mr. Collins was carefully instructing them in what they were to expect, that the sight of such rooms, so many servants, and so splendid a dinner, might not wholly overpower them."

He's right. The thought of any meal with Jane Austen can be a bit overpowering. All that blinding Regency bling: the dining-room tables longer than most of our houses, the glittering platters full of . . . what is that? Peacock!? The bewigged footmen standing guard, paid to look intimidating; the frightful glares of Lady Catherine, who's just noticed you're using the wrong silver spoon to slurp up the turtle soup. Surely none of this is relevant or even sanely replicable in our modern, everyday lives. And I commend you if the thought hasn't already crossed your subconscious mind: *If this book tells me to hire a footman for my health, I'm chucking the ruddy thing out the window!* So, allow me to reassure you in the best Mr. Collins fashion: "Do not make yourself uneasy, my dear cousin." Yes, eating a Jane Austen meal might seem *so 1813* on the surface, but strip away the historic glitz and glamour (nixing the footmen too) and we're left with something remarkably clever underneath. To paraphrase the wisdom of *Persuasion*, three centuries might be enough to change a few menus, spoons, and table manners, but when it comes to the fundamentals of healthy eating, three centuries "may be little more than nothing."

The meals that punctuate every Austen novel have timeless patterns that anyone can replicate (whether you're living in Pemberley or a poky little apartment without a silver anything in sight). You'll even find many of these Regency eating patterns recognizably comfy. Like us, Austen was accustomed to enjoying three meals a day and didn't refuse the occasional snack, but *when* and *how* she ate them defines what she meant by "I eat my meals . . . in a rational way"—a rational meal plan full of sensible reminders for all of us. And it begins, naturally, with breakfast.

"Happy, Happy Breakfast!"

Understanding a proper Regency breakfast first requires understanding what happens "before breakfast" begins—a phrase Austen clearly got good mileage out of:

- Anne and Henrietta explore the seaside at Lyme "before breakfast" in *Persuasion*.
- Bingley travels daily to Longbourn "before breakfast" to see Jane in *Pride and Prejudice*.
- Jane Fairfax regularly walks to the post office "before breakfast" in *Emma*.
- Edward and Elinor enjoy flirty chats "before breakfast" in *Sense and Sensibility*.

There are few sights rarer in Austenworld than somebody doing the opposite: of slumping out of bed and shuffling straight for the breakfast table with incoherent grunts. On the contrary, a definite gap between waking up and eating breakfast was, by far, the Regency norm.[1] A two-hour gap is the usual pattern in Jane's fiction, with her characters normally waking up at 8:00 a.m. but waiting to eat breakfast until 10:00 a.m. The same pattern defined Austen's own morning routine: waking up around 7:00 a.m. and postponing breakfasting until 9:00 a.m.

It goes without saying that Austen characters tend to get an enormous amount accomplished in this "before breakfast" period (shopping, walking, reading, hunting, making us feel like chronic underachievers in comparison). But they also happen to be doing their bodies a tremendous amount of good in the process.

Postponing breakfast for two hours after you wake up is one of the easiest ways to incorporate small, routine "fasts" into your diet. You are, in fact, *supposed* to arrive at breakfast a bit more hungry than usual—a concept literally built into the word itself (i.e., at breakfast we *break our fast*). Austen obviously grasped this historic wisdom. Her "late breakfast" is truly a mini-fast in disguise. Indeed, any time we give our bodies a temporary break from food, we start reaping the known benefits of fasting: a biological repair mode with a slew of miraculous side effects (lowering our cholesterol and blood sugar, burning fat, and regenerating cells). And while you won't find anything as "tiresome" as a forty-day fast in Austenworld (we'll leave that to the creepy hermit who lives in the "hermitage" on the Northanger Abbey estate, thank you very much), Jane's mini-fasts in the morning are still surprisingly effective and far more sane.

As modern health experts now realize, our bodies only need to go about twelve hours without food to enter a state called *negative protein balance*—the cellular repair mode that makes fasting so beneficial. And while you could technically do one of these mini-fasts any time of day, it's unquestionably easiest in the morning.[2] Since you're already sleeping through most of it (eight hours in bed with a normal two-hour break from food before bed), you can easily go twelve hours without eating on Austen's "late breakfast" plan—just the window your body needs to enter its fasting repair mode with full force. Clever Jane.

"No Coffee, I Thank You, For Me"

Austen would have also delayed drinking coffee or tea during her "before breakfast" fast. This was mostly for economic reasons: coffee and tea were expensive commodities in the Regency era and thus reserved until everyone gathered for breakfast. But there's a biological reason to adopt the same practice today. Consumed first thing in the morning, the caffeine in coffee especially can interfere with your body's natural ability to wake up on its own. Caffeine specifically suppresses *cortisol*, the wake-up hormone. Naturally present in the morning, cortisol can get you up and alert faster than any jolt from caffeine. But caffeine, if taken too early, can override cortisol's natural rhythm, making you more tired and more reliant on caffeine to get the same buzz you could have gotten naturally.[3] So do what Austen did—no need to banish coffee from your morning routine: just postpone it for about an hour after rising, enough time for cortisol to work its magic.

As for the type of breakfast Austen recommends, that "is left to your own choice." You are free to enjoy a hearty breakfast—there are eggs and pork on the breakfast table at Mansfield Park—or lighter fare. Most Austenites do prefer lighter breakfasts in general, opting for simple variations on "toast and tea"—the most popular breakfast in the Regency era.

Jane preferred it too. One of her daily morning rituals was toasting the bread and preparing a fragrant pot of tea for her family's breakfast at 9:00 a.m.[4] With a nub of fresh butter and jam or honey to spread over their toast, most Regency eaters were "exceedingly well contented." Most continental Europeans still are: preferring similar coffee-and-croissant combos for their own breakfasts today. Italians have their regular espressos and sugar-dusted croissants, Spaniards their hot chocolates and cinnamon churros. All are reflective of an enduring bit of cross-cultural wisdom: the best time to guiltlessly enjoy your favorite carbs (jammy toast, buttery croissants, etc.) is in the morning, when your body most easily burns those carbs as energy rather than storing them as fat. It should come as no surprise, then, that we only find Jane recommending carb-rich meals within the confines of breakfast.

But whatever breakfast you choose, Jane is clear on one point: you should take a moment to actually *enjoy* it. In Austenworld, rushing through a hasty breakfast is reserved for the odd flight of adventure (such as when Fanny and Edmund have an early-morning carriage to catch in *Mansfield Park*). Otherwise, "a long comfortable breakfast" prevails. Breakfast is such a "favourite meal" for Mrs. Jennings and her daughter in *Sense and Sensibility*, they are evidently peeved when their breakfast party is interrupted—"It must be something extraordinary that could make Colonel Brandon leave my breakfast table so suddenly." Everyone has waited patiently for breakfast; it's now their right to enjoy it.

Channel Mrs. Jennings and reclaim your own right to enjoy breakfast again. Even if it's only for a few moments, taking a midmorning break to relax, unplug, and quietly sip your tea is a "necessary compliment" you owe yourself. Austen doesn't call it "Happy, happy breakfast!" for nothing.

"A Plentiful Dinner"

No, this isn't a typo, and yes, Austen just flagrantly skipped from breakfast to dinner. Wait, whatever happened to lunch? Hmm, I'm sensing another possible book-chucking moment, so let's clarify a few important terms.

What we now call "lunch"—the second main meal of the day served around noon—was unknown to Austen. "Luncheon" for Jane was nothing more than a sort of snack, a rare refreshment eaten between a main meal, if eaten at all (it's why Austen only mentions "luncheon" once, in *Pride and Prejudice*).[5] Dinner was equally different for Jane. Not the evening affairs we know today, but the next main meal directly after breakfast, served around midafternoon. Regency "dinners" are actually closer to what we would call a large, late lunch.

Understanding why any of this matters is crucial to unlocking one of Austen's healthiest eating strategies. After all, Jane viewed dinner exactly how we do today, as "our grand meal" of the day. Regency dinners might involve a few extra and elaborate dishes (with at least "two courses," screams Mrs. Bennet), but the basic premise remains the same. Like us, Austen and her contemporaries were culturally accustomed to eating more at dinner than at any other meal.

The big difference, however, is *when* they ate it. The Bennets sit down to dinner around 4:30 p.m. in *Pride and Prejudice*. The Dashwoods eat their dinner thirty minutes earlier in *Sense and Sensibility*, as do the Woodhouses in *Emma*. Mr. Woodhouse has a positive "horror" of dining any later than that—a feeling Austen clearly sympathized with. "A reasonable dinner hour" always meant an early one for Austen, rarely stretching beyond 5:00 p.m. Those who dine later in her novels are usually a bad or dubious lot (like Henry's lavishly corrupt uncle in *Mansfield Park* and his "accustomary late dinner-hour"). No doubt Austen was thinking of the Prince Regent, the era's poster boy for fashionably late dinners. Feasting at the Prince's palace started at 6:00 p.m. and often dragged on until 10:00 p.m.[6] Sticking to older habits, however, Jane and her family ate their own dinner at 3:30 p.m. in 1798. Ten years later she was still embracing the general concept, writing to her sister: "an early dinner . . . is exactly what we propose."

Eating, as Jane says, your "heartiest meal" earlier in the day is what most of humanity has always proposed. Afternoon dinners were the preferred norm from Roman times to the Middle Ages—a preference that continued well into the Victorian era. Literature buffs will certainly have noticed: the second sentence of *Jane Eyre* states that Mrs. Reed, the housekeeper, "dined early," and Nelly in *Wuthering Heights* won't consider serving dinner any later than "one o'clock."[7] Many modern-day Brits (especially in northern England) still cling to the custom, calling their afternoon meal "dinner" instead of lunch. The same goes for diners in France, Spain, Germany, and most of Europe, for that matter—all preferring to eat their "heartiest meal" in the afternoon at lunch rather than in the evening at dinner.

Nothing could be more sensible, especially for weight control. Closest to the Regency concept of "dinner," a large European-style lunch is undeniably healthier than a large American-style dinner for two reasons. First, filling up on a large, late lunch cleverly solves the modern problem of *afternoon munchies*—that dreaded 3:00 to 4:00 p.m. hunger gap when some of our worst food choices are made. Second, eating your biggest meal earlier in the day gives your body ample time to digest and work off that substantial influx of calories before bed. The alternative: going to sleep on a dinner-laden stomach sets you up for an unnecessary battle with biology since your metabolism naturally slows down at night. Night-shift workers with late eating habits have a substantially increased risk of obesity for this very reason.[8]

Austen was evidently in tune with this biological truth, serving "large dinners" early enough to allow her characters time for "after dinner" activities long before they retire to bed. Indeed, most of the "afternoon" scenes in Jane's novels—the walks to Meryton, the chats over tea, the carriage joy-rides—actually take place in the early evening hours "after dinner." Notice that after dining with the Palmers in *Sense and Sensibility*, Marianne "calculated" that she still has enough time and daylight to for "going out again" for a postprandial walk around the garden.

It's the perfect calculation to remember today. Because while the arrangements of modern life might make Austen's preferred dinner times impractical (except, perhaps, on the weekends), the general "head and heart" of her rule still applies. Enjoy your largest meal earlier in the day and always leave room for an "after dinner" life after dinner.

Replicating a Regency Dinner

Control. In contrast to the modern practice of plating up food (with preset portion sizes) in the kitchen, Regency diners had far more control. Their dinners were served à la française—in the French manner—meaning all the dishes were arranged on the table at once, in what we would now call "family-style" dining. They then helped themselves to the surrounding food, choosing exactly how much (or how little) *they* wanted to eat, not how much their cooks wanted to give them.[9] In Austenworld, you are your "own master" at the table.

Talk. Austen is emphatic: the best dinners come with a large helping of conversation. In the boisterous dinner scene in *Pride and Prejudice*, there are at least six people talking at once, some "in a voice rather louder than" others. "Noise" and "talk" are dinnertime standards in Austenworld, where people gather 'round the table "for the sake of eating, drinking, and laughing together"— and not just for the food. Though we've momentarily forgotten the secret in our rushed, TV-dinner culture, anyone who has gone on a blind date will still recognize Austen's intuitive logic: that people naturally eat less when they talk more.

Dessert. In Austenworld, you have one chance to eat dessert if you want it: *immediately* after dinner. As Jane explains in *Emma*, Regency desserts were seamlessly joined to the end of dinner itself—"the dinner passed away; the dessert succeeded." Postponing dessert with the modern "Oh, I'm too full now, perhaps later" line was unheard of, and clearly not as smart. After a full dinner, you're much more likely to treat dessert with natural moderation, with room enough to indulge in only a few bites. The more you delay dessert, however, the hungrier you'll become, and the bigger your dessert portions are likely to be.[10]

"Let Her Name Her Own Supper"

If you've been crunching the numbers, nervously counting down the long hours between an early Regency dinner and next day's late breakfast, *do not give way to useless alarm*—Jane would never let her characters go to bed hungry. Enter supper, the last element of Austen's meal plan.

Supper was to Jane what a light, late dinner is to us. Quite a small meal, yet still incredibly important to the happiness of her characters. In *Emma*, she makes the wonderfully sassy observation that a long day "without sitting down to supper, was pronounced an infamous fraud upon the rights of men and women."

Suppers were integral at Regency balls (where early dinners and all that dancing inevitably worked up some ravenous evening munchies), but suppers were equally cherished at home. Usually some warm, dainty nibbles brought into the drawing room on a tray, everyone looks forward to "a little bit of hot supper" in Jane's novels. In *Pride and Prejudice*, the promise of a cozy supper after an evening of card games at Mrs. Phillips' house "was very cheering" to all the Bennet girls. It certainly proves the highlight of Mr. Collins' night. He spends the carriage ride home "enumerating all the dishes at supper." And who can blame him? There's something delightfully comforting and reassuring about Regency suppers—Austen's guiltless permission to wind down the long day with a relaxing meal. No wonder Mr. Bingley "scarcely needed an invitation to stay [for] supper."

But are suppers still healthy today?

Jane is very careful on this point: In Austenworld, you have the "right" to eat supper *only* if you've eaten an early dinner. As Jane explains in a personal footnote to her sister, the only reason the Bennets regularly eat supper in *Pride and Prejudice* is because they've kept up the "old . . . habits" of dining early. Otherwise, Austen says, "there might as well have been no suppers at Longbourn" at all. She repeats the rule in *Mansfield Park*. When traveling prevents them from eating an early dinner, Fanny and Edmund have only *one* evening meal at an inn instead: "a comfortable meal, uniting dinner and supper."

Doing so, Austen prevents her characters from falling into an unhealthy pattern: eating two meals too close together, especially too late into the night. For Jane, common sense dictated that people should never go to bed starving, but neither should they have too much food wobbling around in their stomachs. English doctors agreed. Remarking on the best time to go to bed, the seventeenth-century physician Stephen Bradwell said, "Let it be two houres . . . after supper"[11]—a figure remarkably on track with the food-before-sleep time frame still prescribed by modern dieticians.

The same historical wisdom underlines Austen's next supper rule: the later it gets, the lighter your meal should be. "Light suppers make long lives," goes an old English proverb[12]—a dictum reflected throughout Austen's fiction. Remember that Mrs. Phillips only promises "a little bit of hot supper" in *Pride and Prejudice*, not a gargantuan meal. Every Austenite knows that suppers are not, and should never be, in the same "plentiful" league as early dinners. In *Emma*, the Woodhouses help their guests to a few dainty dishes at supper—some "minced chicken," some "scalloped oysters," and "a *little* bit of tart—a *very* little bit." It's a happy, satisfying meal served beside the cozy fireplace at Hartfield, but "little" servings rule the occasion. Elsewhere, Jane describes the supper at Sir John's ball in *Sense and Sensibility* in similar tiny terminology—as "a *mere* sideboard collation"—some refreshments to nibble on between a dance, but nothing more. Lady Middleton (vapidly ignorant as usual) might think this supper too stingy and "did not approve." But that's exactly the point. Stick with "little" and "mere" quantities and you're always free to enjoy "a late supper" with your pals at Pemberley.

"Soup too! Bless Me!"

Nothing screamed *"Supper!"* quite like soup in the Regency era. In *Pride and Prejudice*, Mr. Bingley can't even send out invitations to his ball/supper party at Netherfield until his cook has made enough soup for the occasion. In *Emma*, Miss Bates chooses soup—of all the dishes on the supper table at the Highbury ball—to attack first: "Soup too! Bless Me! I should not be helped so soon, but it smells most excellent, and I cannot help beginning." Austen herself often curled up with a comfortable bowl of soup after late nights out, writing in 1813: "we were home again [after an evening at the theatre] . . . had soup and wine and water, and then went to our holes." You'll find the same rationale behind the popularity of modern soup diets. Being mostly liquid, soup isn't energy dense, which makes it the perfect food for nighttime feeding (a time when you should always be avoiding heavy foods in the first place). Soup is also eaten much slower than other foods, making it more likely to satisfy your evening cravings than other easily-scarfed-down snacks.[13] Regency soups were particularly satisfying in this regard, especially the creamy "white soup" served at the Netherfield ball in *Pride and Prejudice*. (See recipe at the end of the chapter.)

THE JANE AUSTEN DIET

"Nuncheon"

If you want to score some gloating points at your next Austen trivia night, ask everyone what the word *nuncheon* means, as in Willoughby's line from *Sense and Sensibility*: "I left London this morning at eight o'clock, and the only ten minutes I have spent out of my chaise since that time procured me a *nuncheon* at Marlborough." Most readers gloss over the word (or, given its place in Willoughby's final confession speech, assume it involves some sort of stern talking-to from a catholic nun—he deserves it, the cad!). But nuncheon is, in fact, meal related. More precisely, it explains what Austen characters do if they ever get hungry *between* meals. Nuncheon is a Regency snack.

But let's proceed with "friendly caution" here: Austen lived in an age when regular *snacking* (and even the word itself) was totally unknown. Before the modern convenience of packaged snacks and sugary drinks, "grazing" between meals would have been an odd and difficult concept to imagine.[14] Every eating scene in Jane's novels, therefore, almost always takes place within the structured confines of her three main meals: breakfast, dinner, and supper. At all other times, Austen's daily rule of thumb runs thus: nothing "shall ever pass my lips" in between.

But as I promised in the introduction, Jane isn't a bossy boot camper. She wasn't "fond of being starved" and never forces her characters to go too long without eating either. She does "make allowances" when daily life isn't going as planned. Austen knew that the Regency practice of skipping from breakfast to an early dinner could—if not spaced out correctly—leave somewhat of a potential hunger gap around noon. We find Jane Fairfax experiencing exactly this in *Emma*. Eating very little at breakfast, "about the middle of the day [Jane] gets hungry," says Miss Bates.

Which brings us back to nuncheon. Clarifying its timing and purpose, Austen occasionally spells it "noonchine"—in other words, a light refreshment taken around noon. The word *nuncheon* actually evolved into, and was used simultaneously with, the word *luncheon* during Austen's lifetime. But it still meant a midday snack (eaten infrequently) and not an established meal. Dr. Samuel Johnson, whom Austen admired, famously defined lunch in small, snack-like terms: being "as much food as one's hand can hold."[15]

Hence Lydia's "luncheon" in *Pride and Prejudice* is technically a nuncheon, a midday break for refreshment at a roadside inn during Lizzie's journey home from London. There's cold meat and a cucumber salad, says Lydia, but the words she uses to describe this noontime snack—"surprise" and "treat"—prove just how rarely it occurs in Austenworld. Willoughby's "nuncheon" in *Sense and Sensibility* is almost identical. It's a quick snack of "cold beef" and beer—lasting "only ten minutes"—on a day when his normal dining schedule is obviously being interrupted by a long day of travel (and a guilty conscious over Marianne). Yet these are the only references to either "nuncheon" or "luncheon" in Austen's novels—a mark of how incredibly snack-cautious she was. In other words, the only real grazers in Austenworld are the "eight cows" on the Abbey-Mill Farm in *Emma*. Though understanding *why* snacking is not a "daily habit" in Austenworld requires understanding a natural process Austen knew nothing about.

"In Blood and Understanding"

Jane's cautious views on snacking boils down to the secrets in "a few drops of blood." We know it as *insulin*, a hormone secreted in our bloodstream almost every time we eat. Insulin plays an important, healthy role in how we metabolize food: it transforms the sugars from our meal and helps us "burn" them as instant energy. It also processes the sugars we can't use immediately and stores the rest as fuel to burn up later (mostly in the form of body fat). It's a process full of good intentions: all that stored body fat is meant to be burned up later. But as Jane would say, you can easily get "on the wrong side" of insulin.

By eating too often or snacking too frequently, your bloodstream is practically pumping insulin around the clock. You are keeping your "blood sugar" up—true—but you're also keeping your body from performing a crucial function. That is, burning body fat is virtually impossible while insulin is activated after meals (or sugary drinks). Like a biological switch, insulin turns on your body's natural fat-storing mode, a mode that keeps you fueled from instant sugar energy while converting the rest into fat, something that doesn't stop until insulin levels subside.[16] The only sensible trick, of course, is to do what came naturally to Austen before the rise of modern snacking habits. Simply limit how many insulin spikes your body experiences throughout the day, giving your system time to switch back into fat-burning mode before your next meal. Those "low blood-sugar" feelings between meals are normal and positive indicators that your body is getting the chance to switch from sugar fuel to fat fuel.[17] As Jane recognized, these are important times to take advantage of throughout the day for keeping one's body-fat balance in daily check. Insulin, you see, is a bit like Lydia Bennet. It could do with a few less jiggling jumps from time to time.

White Soup for a Netherfield Ball

Serves 8

"As for the ball, it is quite a settled thing, and as soon as Nicholls has made white soup enough, I shall send round my cards."
—Mr. Bingley, *Pride and Prejudice*

A richly flavored broth delicately thickened with cream and ground almonds, white soup steamed with liquid elegance at Regency balls. And it turns out Mr. Bingley is right: made in advance, the soup is even tastier after a day or two resting in the fridge.

INGREDIENTS

1 large onion	8 cups chicken broth
2 celery stalks	1 ½ cups almond flour
4 chicken thighs	1 cup heavy cream
5 bacon slices	Salt, to taste

1. Cut the onion and celery into quarters (they'll be scooped out later). Put them in a large pot with the chicken thighs and whole bacon slices. Pour in the chicken broth.

2. Bring the pot to a boil over high heat; cover and reduce heat to medium-low. Simmer the broth for 2 hours.

3. Using a slotted spoon, remove the cooked chicken thighs to a plate and set aside to cool. Then remove the bacon, onion, and celery from the broth and either discard or nibble on if feeling peckish.

4. Stir the almond flour into the broth. Cover and simmer for another 30 minutes.

5. While the soup is cooking, remove the meat from the chicken thighs (leaving the meat in elegant chunks, not shredding). Set aside.

6. When the broth has finished simmering, remove from the heat and stir in the heavy cream. If needed, season to taste with salt (not black pepper—it will ruin the whiteness). Serve with a flourish of chicken meat garnished on top.

"She had only to rise . . . creeping slowly up the principal staircase, pursued by the ceaseless country-dance, feverish with hopes and fears, soup and negus, sore-footed and fatigued, restless and agitated, yet feeling, in spite of everything, that a ball was indeed delightful."
—*Mansfield Park*

AUSTEN EATS: SUGAR

Oh, dear. Mr. Woodhouse is party-pooping again . . .

It's the Westons' wedding day in *Emma*, and everyone is making merry with a slice of sugary cake—apparently a village-wide health hazard, according to Mr. Woodhouse. All that sugar is "unwholesome," "unfit," and he earnestly tries "to dissuade them from having any wedding cake at all." When that doesn't work, he calls in his personal diet coach (Mr. Perry) to back him up.

Well, err, um . . . "wedding cake *might* certainly disagree with many," says Mr. Perry appeasingly, not wanting to lose his job, poor man. But that doesn't stop the "strange rumor" from circulating. Later that day, all the little Perry children have been mysteriously "seen with a slice of Mrs. Weston's wedding cake in their hands," though "Mr. Woodhouse would never believe it."

The whole scene is only a few sentences long—a comical beginning to a romance comedy—yet Austen's entire (and quite serious) attitude to sugar is woven brilliantly within. Because unlike Mr. Woodhouse—and the party poopers today with their calls to ban sugar from our lives completely—Jane never dreamed of living without the "sweets of pleasure." *Sweet* being a particularly favorite adjective for Austen, she uses it over a hundred times in her novels. But then again, she kept her wits about her too.

"Sense and sweetness" were two sides of the same coin for Jane, recognizing that a smart and happy life is best with a little bit of both. By all modern definitions, Austen was on a remarkably sensible sugar diet without ever being consciously aware of the fact. Her intake of sugar was dramatically less than that of the average American today: a whopping 75 percent less.[1] And yet you won't find a hint of sugary deprivation in her novels. Consider Mrs. Weston's wedding cake. Austen takes evident pleasure in telling us that every last crumb was eaten and fully enjoyed. Despite Mr. Woodhouse's protests, "still the cake was eaten . . . all gone."

Could Austen seriously hold both views in her head at once—essentially keeping to her sugar diet and eating her cake too? *"Yes, and I hope to engage you to be serious likewise."* Here's how she pulled it off:

"With Lock And Key"

The best way to appreciate Austen's unique relationship with sugar is to start with the obvious fact: Jane kept her sugar locked up. Yes, we're talking Fort Knox–style lockdown with sugar kept in a secured "closet" in her house.[2] Trust me, this isn't as wacky as it sounds. Everybody in the Regency era did it. Frankly, that *we* don't do the same today—that we now buy bags of sugar more cheaply than dirt and keep large bowls of it handy on our countertops—would have been difficult for any Regency person to comprehend.

Fact is, sugar in Austen's England was still a "great luxury," more like a delicious spice to be doled out in careful quantities. Sugar was exotic, coming from faraway places in Asia and across the Atlantic (Sir Thomas owns a sugar plantation on the island of Antigua in *Mansfield Park*), and that made it expensive. Not unaffordable, but pricey enough for Jane to get palpably excited over the following anecdote. In 1808, her brother Charles (fighting in the English navy against Napoleon) had captured a French schooner near Bermuda—a valuable "prize," as Austen says, all because it was richly "laden with sugar."

Needless to say, no one wanted to be parted from this so-called "white gold" once they got it, hence the habit of keeping sugar under lock and key (safe from the sticky fingers of Regency servants). But sugar's high price tag also put natural limits on how much everyone consumed. The figures are astounding. At the end of the eighteenth century, Austen and her English contemporaries were eating roughly twenty pounds of sugar per person a year.[3] That might seem substantial, but it's incredibly low when put into modern context. By the early twenty-first century, even the most conservative estimates held that Americans were consuming a gut-punching ninety pounds of sugar per person a year.[4]

I've even done the math here (a rare and wild thing, mind you, math and I being congenital enemies): Austen's average sugar consumption, twenty pounds per year, comes out to only six teaspoons of added sugar per day. A

Eureka! moment if I've ever had one: six teaspoons of total sugar per day is the exact, safest figure now recommended by both the World Health Organization and the American Heart Association. In contrast, most Americans now consume over twenty teaspoons of sugar a day.[5]

"So Much Trash And Sweet Things"

Science has gradually noticed what Mary Musgrove from *Persuasion* recognized back in 1817: If overindulged "to such a degree . . . sweet things" have a dreadful habit of making us "sick." Biologically sick, that is. Sugar isn't metabolized like other foods. Whether it's a spoonful of white sugar, brown sugar, honey, agave nectar, or high-fructose corn syrup, all "sugar" acts basically the same way in our bodies. About half of it heads straight to the liver to be processed (rather like alcohol). The liver does its best to convert the sugar into energy, but it gets overwhelmed very quickly. The equivalent of a couple of pieces of fruit (or less than a can of soda) is about as much sugar energy as your liver can store at any given time. The rest must go somewhere. Most gets transformed into a less flattering form of energy: fat.

For obvious reasons, converting sugar into fat isn't the healthiest process for your body to perform too frequently (there's a reason why modern sugar consumption and obesity rates have surged simultaneously). But there are less obvious reasons too. As with alcohol, too much sugar being constantly processed by your liver can create some outstandingly negative side effects: fattening the liver, type II diabetes, high cholesterol, and heart disease from the increased fatty triglycerides in your blood. High-sugar diets can even wreck your "natural bloom," to use a Regency expression. Excess sugar creates harmful byproducts in your body called "advanced glycation end products" (AGEs for short), causing, appropriately enough, accelerated aging of your skin.[6]

Even Regency doctors grasped the tricky "reality of sweetness," noting the specific reality of "sugar sickness" (an old term for diabetes) whenever their patients' dependence on sweets got out of control. Which explains Mr. Perry's "intelligent" response to the wedding-cake controversy in *Emma*. With medical textbook accuracy, he acknowledges that the sugary "cake might certainly disagree with many—perhaps most people, unless taken moderately."

Unless taken moderately—the solution satisfies the strictest dieter in Austenworld, Mr. Woodhouse. And it's still the most accurate solution today. Nobody can give up sugar completely. Nor do we need to. Sugar has always been a natural fact and pleasure of life. Our bodies have no problem handling it in moderation, a biological knack we've inherited from our prehistoric ancestors who certainly didn't pass up the rare treat of a beehive dripping with honey when they saw it. Austen saw sugar in much the same way.

She lived in an age when sugar (in any form) was still regarded as a special treat to enjoy when the occasion arises. At Mrs. Weston's wedding, for example, everyone guiltlessly helps themselves to a "rich" slice of cake for the simple reason that it *is* special. No one in Austenworld eats this way all the time. Quite the opposite, "sweet things" were always surrounded by an aura of specialness for Jane. The random purchase of a Regency dessert was enough to be included in the "important nothings" of her life. "You know how interesting the purchase of a sponge-cake is to me," she wrote her sister in 1808. Conversely, one of the glaring giveaways that Mrs. Elton of *Emma* is "absolutely dissipated" and clearly not from around the respectable parts of Austenworld is that she expects such sugary treats too often and at inappropriate moments. Notice she is "shocked" that refreshments at everyday card parties don't include a heaping bowl of "ice" (ice cream or sorbets) for the players to snack on. She also finds the quantity of "cakes" served rather "poor" and shabby. The "insufferable woman" clearly has her sugar priorities mixed up.

Though to be fair, Austen had an easier time sorting these sugar priorities than we do. The *expense* of Regency sugar made it easier to limit, just as the *cheapness* of modern sugar makes it harder to resist, hence the now normal intake of twenty teaspoons of sugar a day, a near toxic level over three times what Jane was used to. And yet the reality remains. Unless the bizarre or impossible happens (we fall into a time warp, we start locking up our sugar, we capture sugar-laden schooners in Napoleonic sea battles), it doesn't seem like sugar is ever going back to Regency standards. *"'Well,' said the still waiting Harriet . . . 'What shall I do? What would you advise me to do?'"*

"You must take care of yourself," says Jane. And luckily, recreating your own world of Regency sugar sanity is easier than it sounds. Below are the top three strategies Austen would have used to naturally limit her own "sweet dependence" and keep sugar in its safe place: No locks, battles, or time warps needed.

1. "Satisfied with Less"

By far, the easiest way to *decrease* your daily sugar intake is to *increase* your natural sugar sensitivity (i.e., how sweet you prefer your food and drinks). Because what might be normal for us (what we now call "sweet," "too sweet, or "not sweet enough") simply wasn't the same in the Regency era.

Too costly to use carelessly, Jane added sugar to her food and drinks with a purposefully light hand. Our "sugar will last a great while," says Austen, congratulating herself on how careful she's been with stretching her family's supply. The practice was so common, it gave nearly everyone in the Regency era a much more heightened sense of sweetness than what we're used to today. In fact, the now acceptable sweetness of modern desserts (and even "savory" foods like mustards, pickles, and salad dressings) would have certainly fallen into the *too sweet,* or even repulsive, category for most Regency eaters.[7] The good news, however, is that you can easily recalibrate your personal sugar sensitivity to these historically heightened levels.

Researchers have found that sweetness is a fluid concept. The less sugar people eat, the better they become at tasting it.[8] Essentially, you can train your taste buds to be, as Austen says, "satisfied with less." Try it out on your next cup of coffee or tea. Take away a small, barely perceptible amount of sugar from the amount you're generally used to (⅛ teaspoon should work). Give your taste buds a few days to get used to the new level of sweetness, then repeat the process again, taking away another ⅛ teaspoon and waiting a few days to adjust. Continue until you reach "astonishment . . . beyond expression" at how much sugar you've cut from your diet without ever feeling deprived.

2. "Conceal Nothing"

Austen lived in a world that was totally upfront and honest with its sugar use. In other words, Jane *knew* when she was eating sugar; it was almost *only* added to foods that were *supposed* to be sweet: desserts, jams, cakes, etc. And while you might think the same logic applies today, things are not as straightforward anymore.

We now live in a world with far more "secrecy and concealment," as they say in *Emma*. Sugar lurks in practically everything with a nutrition label, in foods that have never needed added sugar in the first place (a consequence of the low-fat craze of the 1990s when food companies, pressured out of using fat, added the only flavorful alternative: sugar).

This now means that your *low-fat* yogurt often contains more sugar than a can of soda. Or that certain brands of tomato sauce have more sugar in one serving than the equivalent of a chocolate chip cookie. Or that modern sandwich bread has almost a teaspoon of added sugar in each slice.

Even foods advertised as "no sugar added" are usually hiding a sweeter-than-you-think secret, slyly using concentrated fruit juice (still sugar!) as a loophole. Today, 80 percent of our packaged foods contain added sugar,[9] making us far more likely to zoom past Austen's safe sugar speed limit (six teaspoons) before even reaching dessert.

Which is why we should all be reading those nutrition labels for the same reason Catherine Morland reads boring history books: "I read [them] a little as a duty." They may not be as titillating as *The Mysteries of Udolpho*, but it's our duty to find out how much sugar is concealed within. And if the number is too high for Regency comfort (bearing in mind that four grams of sugar equals one teaspoon), choose more natural alternatives with less hyperactive sugar contents. *"In short, put an end to the miserable state of concealment that has been carrying on so long."*

3. "So Valuable a Fruit"

You'd be hard pressed to find a sugar craving in Austenworld that isn't, in some way, satisfied with fruit. Baked apples are a favorite treat of Jane Fairfax in *Emma*—"there is nothing she likes so well as these baked apples," says

Miss Bates, prompting the most long-winded ode to apples in English literature. Then there's the "cake" served to Lizzie at Pemberley, duly accompanied by "the finest fruits in season . . . beautiful pyramids of grapes, nectarines, and peaches." In *Sense and Sensibility*, a basket full of fruit is one of the first housewarming gifts the Dashwoods receive from Sir John—a sweet pick-me-up after their long journey.

Like General Tilney in *Northanger Abbey*, most everybody in the Regency era "loved good fruit." Indulging in a decadent and overly sugary "dessert course" after dinner simply wasn't the everyday custom. Instead, most members of Austen's class preferred a platter of fresh fruit and nuts to finish off the meal,[10] plucked straight from the garden when available. When not in season, then some sort of pastry made with fruit preserves (like the "apple tarts" served at Hartfield) would satisfy. There was a definite penny-pinching element in all of this (relying on the natural sweetness of nature was cheaper than buying sugar itself), but health played a role too.

Interestingly, the only time Austen uses the word "wholesome" to describe anything sweet is when fruit is involved. Miss Bates even calls her baked apples "extremely wholesome"—albeit somewhat exaggeratingly. The woman is excessively fond of stretching facts; and the fact remains that the sugar naturally found in fruit is *technically* no healthier than regular table sugar. But Miss Bates is on the right track. Fruit has one thing regular sugar doesn't have: a "wholesome" little thing called fiber.

Fiber is to sugar what money is to a Regency marriage—it moves things along rather nicely. Being the indi-
gestible bits of plants, fiber slows down the digestion of
whatever food is eaten alongside of it—sugar included.
Whereas sugar itself is absorbed quickly in your body,
creating the fast sugar spikes so potentially toxic to your
biology, sugar eaten with fiber (a.k.a. fruit) is much more
slowly absorbed. Like a sponge, fiber swells and traps the
sugar in your intestines before slowly releasing it to your
liver. Not only is this gentler on the liver, absorbing sugar
slowly allows your body more time to burn it off as energy
rather than storing it as fat.

Nature cleverly reflects this principle. All fruits contain
fiber, the only sugary treats with built-in safety breaks.
Jane evidently picked up on this natural cue. Sugar highs
in Austenworld only come in the form of "wholesome"
fruit, the midsummer strawberry feast in *Emma* being
the best example. In it, everyone tickles their sweet tooth
with guiltless abandon—"strawberries, and only strawberries, could now be thought or spoken of. 'The best fruit
in England—everybody's favorite—always wholesome.'"
But the scene also hints at the dual secret of eating sugar
with fiber—it fills you up faster and more effectively than
sugar alone. Which is exactly what happens to the strawberry stuffers in *Emma*. They soon experience the sugar
safety breaks of nature. The strawberries may be "delicious," they all say, but admittedly "too rich to be eaten
much of."

"Be It Sweetness or Be It Stupidity"

If you're thinking of skirting around Austen's sugar limits with artificial sweeteners, *"she begged him to think again on the subject."* Not invented until the twentieth century, those little pink, blue, and yellow packets (all promising sweetness without the calories) would have never entered Jane's wildest dieting dreams. And it's just as well we eliminate them from our diets too. Scientific suspicions have always surrounded these zero-calorie sweeteners, especially their claims for helping us lose weight. But new research suggests they might actually be doing the opposite. Artificial sweeteners seem to negatively affect the balance of good bacteria in our gut—the helpful microbes so important for keeping our digestion and metabolism in check.[11] Which could explain why population studies are now linking the consumption of artificial sweeteners (especially in diet sodas) with weight gain, not weight loss. Though none of this would surprise Jane. Nothing "artificial" is completely trustworthy in Austenworld.

Miss Bates' Wine-Baked Apples

Serves 4

*"There is nothing she likes so well
as these baked apples."*
—Emma

Baking apples in a sweet puddle of wine was a popular technique of the era, resulting in a delicious cross between a poached and baked apple with a syrupy sauce for spooning over later.

INGREDIENTS

2 baking apples (Honeycrisps work well)

2 tablespoons raspberry jam

½ cup fruity white wine, such as Pinot Grigio

2 tablespoons butter, cut into chunks

Whipped cream for serving

Preheat oven to 375°.

1. Peel the apples and cut them in half lengthwise. Scoop out the seeds and core with a spoon and lay the apple halves, flat side down, in a pie pan. Take a small knife and pierce the top of the apples a few times (to allow the wine to seep in better). Set aside.

2. Put the raspberry jam and wine into a large bowl and whisk until well combined. Pour over the apples in the pie pan, lifting each apple to make sure the wine mixture gets underneath as well.

3. Scatter the butter around the apples and bake in the oven, uncovered, for 30 minutes. Remove from the oven, carefully flip the apples over in the pie pan, then return to the oven to cook for another 10 minutes.

4. Serve warm or chilled with fresh whipped cream and a drizzle of the winey juices from the pan.

"Oh! What a sweet little cottage there is among the trees—apple trees, too!"
—*Northanger Abbey*

"Drink a little more,
and you will do very well"

—Emma

4

DRINKS WITH JANE

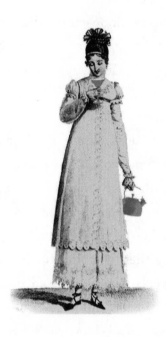

Lovers of alliteration may wonder why I didn't style this chapter, "Drinks with Darcy" or even, "Boozing with Bingley." As in: let's all stumble down to the village tavern where the men of Austenworld are gathered (loosened cravats, riding boots on the table), riveting the crowd with a few macho tips on holding your liquor. For two very good reasons: (a) I'm rather hopeless at imparting macho tips, and (b) the smartest drinking advice doesn't come from Austen's men at all, but from her women.

You'll have to take Jane's word for it. The hearty injunction "Go . . . and drink a little more" comes from one of her female characters; and by and large, it's her women who have figured out how to do just that in the healthiest way possible. Austen's men, on the other hand, usually lag a few wobbly paces behind, some of them quite literally. Like Admiral Croft or Mr. Allen, it's difficult to be a paradigm of *drinking well* when you're dragging a bandaged, bulbous, and gouty leg behind you—a direct consequence of *drinking wrongly*.

Don't get me wrong, Jane wasn't a raving food feminist, but when it comes to hydrating healthfully, it's best to get in touch with your inner Austen heroine (speaking of which, should imagination fail you, wrapping one's shoulders in a makeshift shawl usually works wonders). After all, "to drink their good health" is a loaded expression in Jane's novels, one involving far more secrets than just popping a cork of Madeira. So flagons down and boots off the table, please! This is how real Regency girls quench a "laudable thirst."

"But Indeed I Would Rather Have Nothing But Tea"

Let's start with the go-to beverage, the drink all heroines "should prefer . . . to anything." Find the words *drink* or *drinking* in a Jane Austen sentence and you're almost guaranteed to find a nice cup of tea at the end of it. *Emma* alone has fifteen tea references. *Mansfield Park* has eight.

Coffee? Meh. Cocoa? Nope. "I am much obliged to you . . . but I prefer tea."

It all seems rather quaint and cutesy to us. Ah, tea with Jane Austen—warm fuzzies emanate from the very phrase. But there's more to Jane's "offer of tea" than a few crocheted doilies and pinky-up fingers. In fact, Austen's promotion of tea was practically edgy by Regency health standards.

A relatively new and exotic "leaf" from far-flung China (*leaf* pronounced with a knowing wink and nudge), tea was still regarded as something of a novelty drug to the English. Its side effects were mild but confusing: tea seemed able to simultaneously pep people up and calm them down. No one knew quite what to make of it. Apothecary shops (the pharmacies of the day) were still selling tea as a type of medicine,[1] adding to its mystique and sparking a national debate over the health or harm of this herbal potation.

While some thought it perfectly safe to "sip salubrious tea," many doctors had serious concerns. "The tea pots full of warm water I see upon their tables . . . put me in mind of Pandora's box, from whence all sorts of evils issue forth," wrote the physician Samuel Tissot in 1768, less than a decade before Austen's birth.[2] And the debate continued as Jane attempted her last novel, *Sanditon*.

In it, a character named Arthur Parker believes that drinking tea is tantamount to a trippy drug experience. "It acts on me like poison and would entirely take away the use of my right side before I had swallowed it five minutes

. . . it has happened to me so often than I cannot doubt it. The use of my right side is entirely taken away for several hours!" Given the fact that Mr. Parker is the biggest buffoon in the novel, it's obvious which side of the tea debate Austen was on.

Though despite having no way of scientifically knowing if this exotic brew was healthy or not, Jane spoke up for tea with the tree-stumping passion of a Lorax. Even today, there are few greater tributes to drinking tea than those found in Jane's novels. "Perhaps you would like some tea?" Every smart heroine confidently answers *yes*. The heroine of *Sanditon* even makes a bold prediction: that one day it will be "the simplest thing in the world" to prove the effect tea has on the body—"by those who have studied . . . tea scientifically and thoroughly understand all the possibilities of their action on each other." Meanwhile, Austen reminds her characters to drink up—"You *must* drink tea." It's the closest Jane gets to issuing a dietary command. Turns out she was brilliantly correct.

"In Quest of Tea"

Tea now solidly ranks as one of the healthiest drinks on the planet. Thanks to decades of modern research—*"by those who have studied . . . tea scientifically"*—and thousands of years of human observation (it was already China's national beverage in 350 AD[3]), tea is now the easiest, cheapest, safest, and most potent superdrink in your dieting arsenal.

Important clarification: I'm just talking about regular tea—the dried leaves of the *Camellia sinensis* shrub (the tea plant) steeped in boiling water. The same tea the herbalists of ancient China recognized as the "elixir of life."[4] The same tea Austen eagerly purchased from Twinings in 1814 and pours out so frequently in her novels. The same tea steaming in tubby pots around the world—be it black, green, white, or Earl Grey. The only difference? We now better understand *why* everybody should be, as Jane says, in serious "quest of tea."

Refresh. There's an insightful line in *Mansfield Park* that hints at the first miracle of tea: Fanny quenches her thirst with "a little tea" and it soon "refreshed . . . her body." Science can now confirm that tea literally does just that, refreshing our bodies on a cellular level. Tea contains an abundant source of polyphenols—powerful antioxidants. Polyphenols are nature's protective chemicals, a Molotov cocktail of defense compounds helping plants stay strong by warding off unwanted pests and diseases. Polyphenols do practically the same thing in our bodies whenever we eat (or drink) them, boosting our ability to fight cell damage in our organs, particularly the heart.[5] Red wine has undoubtedly been the polyphenol superstar in recent years (helped along by the cultural phenomenon that some of the world's biggest red winos—the French—have relatively low rates of heart disease). But tea packs an equal polyphenol punch. There are just as many cell-protecting polyphenols in a large mug of tea as in a standard glass of red wine.[6] Which could explain another cultural phenomenon: countries with the highest green tea consumption (such as Japan) have some of the lowest rates of cancer and cardiovascular disease, not to mention equally low obesity rates—another likely power punch from polyphenols. According to research from the University of California, the polyphenols in tea can aid weight loss by acting like prebiotics, encouraging the growth of metabolism-boosting bacteria in our gut.[7] Essentially, tea can help us burn fat without us getting off our bums. Not entirely recommended, but certainly a recognized benefit of tea even back in the eighteenth century. "The proper use [of tea]," wrote Samuel Johnson in 1757, "is to . . . dilute the full meals of those who cannot use exercise."[8] Accordingly, those "who cannot use exercise" in Austenworld cannot seem to live without tea either. The elderly Mrs. Bates, for instance, "was a very old lady, almost past everything but tea."

Soothe. Tea is the "cup that cheers," according to William Cowper, a favorite poet of Austen's, and obviously one of her favorite beliefs about tea. In almost all her novels, tea is a liquid mood booster, magically bringing "comfort" and "content" with every sip. It's the first thing that soothes Catherine's "jaded" spirits after her nightmare at Northanger Abbey; and tea is there to calm Fanny's "head and heart" following her emotional journey from Mansfield

Park—all very accurate observations. Tea is *nootropic*—it literally enhances the way we think. It does this through a special amino acid called L-theanine, one of the few plants in the world with this unique compound. L-theanine relieves tension and anxiety by stimulating alpha-wave patterns in our brains (the brain waves that make us feel both relaxed and mentally focused)[9]—the same patterns stimulated during meditation. In 2004, L-theanine was even found to be more effective at reducing anxiety during relaxation than the modern sedative Xanax,[10] confirming the wisdom of an ancient Chinese poem: "tea . . . banishes my loneliness and melancholy."[11] Austen's England was full of similar findings. In 1763, James Boswell found tea to be "a most kind remedy" whenever he felt depressed, "low-spirited," "dull," and "miserable."[12] Fresh from the trauma of fighting at Waterloo, Captain John Kincaid relied on tea as "the most sovereign restorative of jaded spirits."[13] Three centuries later, most modern Brits would still agree. There's seemingly no trauma in England that can't be made infinitely better by "a nice cup of tea." It's the national knee-jerk reaction for bad breakups, scraped knees, divorces, and general life stress: *Right, then, I'll put the kettle on.* This was spectacularly demonstrated during the London bombings in 2005, when local shopkeepers rushed to the shocked, dazed, and wounded with—what else?—bracing cups of tea. "A Very British Response to Terror," said the *New York Times*.[14] But it was Austen's exact response too. After the stress of

Marianne's near-death experience, Elinor seeks immediate solace in a nice cup of tea—"leaving Marianne still sweetly asleep, she joined Mrs. Jennings in the drawing-room to tea . . . and the present refreshment . . . was particularly welcomed." Clearly, not knowing L-theanine by name (is he related to Lady Dalrymple?) didn't stop Austen from recognizing its happy effects: "Before tea, it was a rather dull affair, but then . . . after tea we cheered up."

Stimulate. Caffeine wasn't technically "discovered" until 1827, though its stimulating power was common knowledge to Jane, hence tea's appearance as the energy drink of Regency balls, coming to the rescue of the exhaustedly twirled about. "Everybody was shortly in motion for tea"— so begins the mad "squeeze" to the tea room at Catherine's first ball in *Northanger Abbey*. But Jane also recognized that tea stimulates rather gently. None of her characters become wired or buzzed after drinking tea, even when taken at night (evening tea drinking is habitual in Jane's novels). Even the most sensitive body in Austenworld, Mr. Woodhouse, can't imagine tea interfering with sleep in the slightest. On the contrary, "You will get very tired when tea is over," he tells Emma. Today, tea is just as gentle on our own bodies, the safest way to get a measured dose of caffeine. A drug by any other name, caffeine comes with some naturally stressful side effects—heart palpitations, hypertension, anxiety—but its presence in tea comes with equally natural safeguards. There's less of it to worry about: even the strongest black teas have half the caffeine of coffee; lighter green teas have one-sixth the amount.[15] Then there's tea's unique chemical makeup: the calming presence of L-theanine naturally counteracts the more unpleasant side effects of caffeine, neutralizing the jitters caffeine would normally induce on its own. You can't say the same for coffee, a drink with far more caffeine without the soothing balance of L-theanine. Interestingly, Austen didn't say much for coffee either. It wasn't a usual beverage in the Austen household, and Miss Bates refuses it outright in *Emma*—"No coffee, I thank you, for me—never take coffee." A wise move. Congenitally high strung, Miss Bates has enough natural jitters to be getting on with. Ergo she'll stick with "a little tea if you please."

Dieticians might even be returning to one of the biggest reasons Austen drank tea in the first place—it was healthier than water. Before modern filtration techniques, Regency water was infamously risky to drink *au naturel*. Austen noticed "dirt" in her water decanter in 1804 and Tobias Smollett, another period novelist, noticed a bit more than that. "If I would drink water, I must quaff the mawkish contents of an open aqueduct, exposed to all manner of defilement . . . impregnated with all the filth of London."[16] This alone made tea an incredible health boon to Austen and her contemporaries: the boiling water required to make tea effectively killed any microbes bobbing within.

And while mass germicide may no longer be our *raison d'être* for putting the kettle on, there's reason enough to swap out a plain glass of water for a nice cup of tea. After studying more than a decade of tea research in 2006, Dr. Ruxton from the *European Journal of Clinical Nutrition* reported her findings to the BBC: "Drinking tea is actually better for you than drinking water. Water is essentially replacing fluid. Tea replaces fluid and contains antioxidants, so it's got two things going for it." The report went on to confirm that tea is just as hydrating as water; the minimal amount of caffeine in tea isn't enough to dehydrate our cells.[17]

However, treating tea like a Regency water cooler is only smart if you're drinking it correctly. And luckily, Jane has a few things to say about how people should "take their tea"—her basic guidelines just as relevant and reliable today.

"Questions Now Eagerly Poured Forth"

How much? At the very least, tea is sipped twice daily in Austenworld: during breakfast and a few hours after dinner (the two normal "tea times" in Jane's novels). Multiple cups were usually consumed at each sitting. Austen herself reckoned that a Regency family would likely go through about twelve pounds of tea every four months—approximately four cups a day. The figure falls exactly in line with Dr. Ruxton's report in the *European Journal of Clinical Nutrition* that drinking three to four cups of tea a day will get you closest to reaping its full polyphenol benefits.[18]

What Type? Austen was an equal opportunity tea drinker, enjoying both black and green tea and rarely differentiating between the two. A smart move. Every tea leaf—whether it's black, green, or white (in a bag or loose leaf)—comes from only one plant, which means all teas share the same basic health benefits. The only difference is in the way the tea leaves are dried, affecting their color and taste. Their antioxidant powers, however, remain relatively identical, with only different *types* of antioxidants in different types of tea.[19] But even Jane seems to have had her preference. A "naturally intelligent" woman would drink "green tea," she wrote in a letter of 1813. Quite a clever observation, actually, because while technically no "healthier" than black tea, green tea is undoubtedly easier to drink in healthier ways (see the next two points below).

Cream? Careful. Jane only admired people who *don't* cream their tea. "There are two traits in her character which are pleasing," she wrote about a new acquaintance in 1796, "namely, she admires Camilla [the novel] and drinks no cream in her tea." This could easily be chalked up to Austen's natural preference for green tea)—a drink (unlike black tea) that isn't usually consumed with cream)—though it's not a bad prejudice to pick up ourselves. Adding cream to tea could reduce its antioxidant benefits (according to a German study in 2007). The proteins in cream or milk can bind with the polyphenols in tea, making it harder for your body to absorb them.[20] More studies are needed to confirm this, but it's probably best to keep cream to a minimum in tea. Or, do an Austen-approved switch from black tea to green.

Sugar? Austen wasn't against adding sugar to tea, but she did view it as something reservedly special)—"and then, the Tea and Sugar!")—her exclamation implying a sweet treat and not an everyday habit. Essentially, Austen wasn't gulping down warm sugar water the whole day through (flip back to the previous chapter for a reminder as to why). Like most modern green-tea drinkers, she probably didn't even need sugar in her daily cup: green tea is famously easy to drink without sugar, being far less bitter and astringent than black tea. But if you find yourself hankering for a cup of sweet, creamed tea (and I personally *adore* an occasional cup myself), it helps to remember one big Regency rule. Keep it small. Jane's porcelain teacups were minuscule by modern standards, holding less than one-half cup of liquid. Modern mugs, by contrast, hold double that amount, therefore requiring double the amount of sugar to sweeten)—a good enough reason to dig out your grandmother's old china teacups from storage. They're the healthiest way to enjoy "a little bit of tea" when you want it a little bit sweet.

"Where the Waters Do Agree"

Now that we've thoroughly praised the kettle, we can move on to the pump. Plain water wasn't exactly a barred Regency beverage, but some "waters" were considered markedly healthier than others. Specifically, the water bubbling up from England's mineral springs had been credited with health-giving properties since the Roman occupation of the island. The Romans founded an entire spa town around one of these springs in southern England, calling it Aquae Sulis. Still thriving at the turn of the nineteenth century, Austen called it Bath.

Every reader of *Northanger Abbey* or *Persuasion* knows about Bath—the Regency hydro resort where the sick and health sapped go to "take the waters." Pouring from a decorative pump just above the natural spring, you're sure to find a friendly face in the elegant "pump room" at Bath. Some are there for serious health reasons, such as Admiral Croft or Mr. Allen, "drinking his glass of water" to relieve his "gouty constitution." Others enjoy it as an added health bonus. Mrs. Elton of *Emma* remembers her mineral water regimen in glowing terms: "Let me recommend Bath to you . . . where the waters do agree, it is quite wonderful the relief they give." Austen herself lived five years in Bath, frequently passing the pump room with its famous inscription etched over the doorway: WATER IS BEST. Meaning, of course, *mineral* water is best. But is it really? Are there modern benefits in becoming, like Anne Elliot, "a person in Bath who drinks the water"?

"The Water Has Been of Use To Her"

To put it in modern terms, the water in *Persuasion*'s pump room was naturally "hard." Hard water, unlike soft water, is rich in natural mineral salts—the stuff that leaves scummy residue in some of our showers, the same stuff that was forever building up on the pump room's pump in Bath—stuff that could have some significant health impacts.

Around the 1970s, scientists in Britain first began noticing an interesting anomaly: people who lived in hard-water regions tended to have less heart disease than their soft-water-drinking neighbors.[21] Recent explanations have centered on magnesium, one of the primary minerals found in hard water. Essential to heart health, magnesium helps regulate our blood pressure, maintains heart rhythms, and (in a reverse blessing to what hard water does to our showers) keeps our arteries clean from plaque buildup. Like most mineral water today, magnesium was part of the chemical makeup of Bath's water; even Austen got incredibly close to realizing its benefits were heart related. "The water" promotes "a better circulation of the blood," she told her sister, repeating the words of an "intelligent" doctor treating her brother in Bath in 1799.

Drinking mineral water is also one of the easier ways to add a valuable bit of magnesium to your diet. Magnesium has always been a tricky mineral to get strictly from food (accounting for why most Americans are now magnesium deficient).[22] So unless you live in a hard-water region, you might want to splash out on the modern equivalent of a trip to Bath—buying the occasional bottle of mineral water. Many European brands have naturally higher magnesium levels (usually listed on their labels) along with other beneficial minerals, including calcium, iron, and potassium. Most contain some of the same forty-two minerals that gurgled out of the pump at Bath,[23] posing the question: Was it really Mr. Tilney or miracle mineral water that made "Catherine hasten to the pump-room the next day" "with more than usual eagerness"?

"A Happy Alternative" to Soda

In case you're still wondering—"she felt it incumbent on her to hint"—soda is not included in the Regency beverage package. Living decades before the first

carbonated soft drinks were mass produced meant
Austen simply made do without them. Which, lucky
for her, meant living without the now number-one
source of empty calories in modern diets[24] (soda is
essentially water with *nine* teaspoons of sugar in each
pop). But Austen didn't go entirely without those pops
and bubbles either. You'll find the refreshing alternative in *Emma*: "spruce beer." The Regency equivalent
of homemade root beer (with an evergreen twist),
spruce beer is a favorite summer drink of both Emma
and Mr. Knightley: "Talking about spruce beer—Oh!
yes—Mr. Knightley and I both saying we liked it." Flavored with the vitamin-rich leaves of the spruce fir,
spruce beer was even considered a "diet drink" by
many doctors. With far less sugar than modern soda,
it is "highly refreshing in summer, and sits easy on
the most debilitated stomach," remarked *A Practical
Treatise on Diet* in 1801.[25] "We are brewing spruce
beer again," said Austen excitedly. Try bubbling up a
batch yourself with the updated recipe at the end of
the chapter.

Tea? Water? Regency pop? *My, what "a continual
supply of the most amiable and innocent enjoyments."*
But when does the alcohol arrive at this Austen party?
Quite right, it was heartless of me to dangle the promise of a few hard drinks at the start of the chapter only
to go soft throughout most of it. I suppose I was pulling

a Mr. Collins: increasing your suspense "according to the usual practice of" infuriating writers. Very wrong of me. So let's have no more delay. Here's what Austen has to say about those "stronger impulses."

"I Hope You Will Drink"

The good news first. Austen was no abstainer. Like most Regency women, alcohol was as much an innocent enjoyment in her life as a nice cup of tea. Jane loved making homemade wines, asking her friends for recipes for "orange wine," and was particularly fond of "mead" brewed fresh from the honey in her sister's beehives. Trips away from home brought other drinking pleasures. One of the definite perks of staying with rich friends and relations, Austen told her sister, was drinking fancy "French wine" every day. Atta girl, Janey!

Her heroines likewise see nothing inherently wrong with alcohol. Emma even advises it for general well-being, coaxing a stressed-out Frank Churchill to take a chill pill with an enlivening glass of Madeira: "Go . . . and drink a little more, and you will do very well . . . another draught of Madeira and water, will make you nearly on par with the rest of us." The feeling is echoed by the women of *Sense and Sensibility*. A "glass of wine" makes a heartbroken Marianne "more comfortable," and Mrs. Jennings soon prescribes another dose of the liquid anodyne: "I have just recollected that I have some of the finest old Constantia wine in the house that was ever tasted, so I have brought a glass of it for your sister." This time Elinor swigs the wine herself, as much in need of "its healing powers" as Marianne.

So far, Austen is on the right track. The "healing powers" of alcohol have been well documented over the years, with study after study confirming the common benefits. Alcohol reduces your risk of developing heart disease or suffering an ischemic stroke (severe reduction of blood flow to the brain), and increases your level of HDL (good) cholesterol. But there's one equally common catch. Only *moderate* consumption of alcohol can impart these body benefits: currently understood as one drink a day for women and no more than two drinks a day for men. Go over that amount and you quickly transform a health tonic into, as Austen would say, a "sad poison." Literally everything reverses—your risk of stroke, heart disease, "bad" cholesterol, cancer, and liver damage all go up as your alcohol consumption exceeds the moderate limit.[26] Intoxication has the word *toxic* in it for good reason. A warning well understood by 1750: "an immoderate use of strong liquors imbecilitates the human body," reported a lady's magazine that year.[27]

"I Fear for His Liver"

It further explains why Jane played it so careful with alcohol, doling out authorial wrist slaps whenever her characters overdo it. The mere mention of binge drinking gets a firm reprove in *Pride and Prejudice*. "If I were as rich as Mr. Darcy," boasts one of the stupider Lucas boys, "I would . . . drink a bottle of wine a day." Mrs. Bennet fires back: "Then you would drink a great deal more than you ought . . . and if I were to see you at it, I should take away your bottle directly."

Pity Mrs. Bennet wasn't patrolling the neighborhood of Mansfield Park. Tom Bertram wrecks his body and almost dies from "a good deal of drinking." The same "dirty and gross" habit destroying Fanny's father. He drinks like a sailor and wafts a "smell of spirits" wherever he goes, constantly "calling out for his rum and water." "I fear for his liver," says a character in *Sanditon*, speaking of another bibulous gent, Arthur Parker—a man who's not only wrong about tea, he's wrong about alcohol too. "The more wine I drink . . . the better I am," says Arthur, the girth of his "heavy" wine belly proving it. And though we don't know what ultimately becomes of his drinking habits (Austen never finished *Sanditon*), the early prognosis isn't promising. Poor Arthur hovers "at the point of death" even at the start of the story.

You may have noticed the masculine thread running through these examples. Bad drinkers in Austenworld are *all* men. You'll never find her female characters tippling out of proportion, let alone getting wasted. Even party girl Lydia Bennet gets higher on giggles than on alcohol. The unwritten rules of Regency respectability kept "the gentle sex" in a much gentler relationship with booze. Two of their top rules can even help keep our own attitude toward alcohol in check today.

1. "The Grossest Falsehood!"

Regency men were famous for falling for the same zinger most of us fell for in college—that drinking is somehow cool, and overdrinking even cooler. John Thorpe, Austen's obnoxious frat boy in *Northanger Abbey*, has fallen for it completely. He brags to Catherine about drinking "his bottle a day" and shrugs off the ten cups of wine chugged at his "last party" at Oxford as nothing very "remarkable." He waits for her to swoon into his inebriated arms. She never does. No Austen heroine can stomach it.

Drinking to excess is repulsively dweeby to them, one of the quickest turn-offs in Austenworld. For Emma, friendly Mr. Elton transforms into an instant creep the minute she suspects "he had been drinking too much of Mr. Weston's good wine." A "swelling resentment" defines their relationship from there on. For Elinor, Willoughby hits an all-time smarmy low by just joking about being "in liquor." "Yes, I am very drunk," he scoffs, though he might just have well screamed, "and I have syphilis too!" for the disgust on Elinor's face. Like seducing hapless women, there's an element of selfishness in getting drunk that Austen always despised. Which is why more "delicate—tender—truly feminine" enjoyment of alcohol is far more about thinking of *others* in her novels.

Darcy, for one, really makes Lizzie swoon by offering alcohol for *her* relief, not his. Responding "in a tone of gentleness" after Lizzie receives bad news about Lydia, Darcy is all kindness and concern: "Is there nothing you could take to give you present relief?" he says. "A glass of wine; shall I get you one?" Edmund acts the same heroic bartender in *Mansfield Park*, bringing a reviving "glass of Madeira to Fanny" after her exhausting day with Mrs. Norris. All said, drinking alcohol without bringing comfort to others is "a very flat business" in Austenworld. The worst wine being "wine drank without any smiles."

2. "Inventing Excuses"

Etiquette played an even larger role in keeping Austen heroines in a safe relationship with alcohol. During normal Regency dinners, wine was only brought out with the dessert course—"when the dessert and the wine were arranged," as Austen says in *Sense and Sensibility*. Ladies would enjoy their glass of wine (usually just one) and then promptly "withdraw" from the table, leaving the menfolk behind.[28] The actual logic for this was rather silly and blatantly sexist—i.e., the men had been on their best "ladies are present" behavior throughout dinner, and now the poor dears needed some time to relax, toss up a few bawdy jokes, and tease Wickham about his latest tart. "No, no, Mr. Collins, the *other* sort of tart!" Ribald laughter ensuing.

But it's the women who got the last laugh. While they were satisfied with their one-and-done glass of wine after dinner, the men who lingered behind also lingered over the bottle. The "general rate of drinking," as Mr. Thorpe reminds us, was astonishing. Left to their own devices, Regency men could easily polish off two bottles of wine apiece after dinner.[29] Diarists of the time recorded even more epic examples: like the liver-pulverizing dinner party described by Sylas Neville in the late 1700s—where ten men went through "27 bottles of claret and 12 of port, besides punch, and were all beastly drunk."[30] Ya think?! But even Dr. Grant, the supposed holy man of *Mansfield Park*, knows these occasions as automatic excuses for drinking. Having Henry Crawford as a permanent guest at his dinner table means only one thing to Dr. Grant: "an excuse for drinking claret every day"—one of the many lifestyle "excuses" that effectively kills him by the end of the novel.

Austen's takeaway here is timeless: "inventing excuses" for overdrinking never ends well. Drinking "because the ladies have left the table" has now morphed into "because it's the weekend!" or "because it's a party!" or "because I finally got the kids to bed, woop!"—all of which will quickly transform alcohol from a tonic to a toxin in your body. Better to vicariously leave the table with the ladies of Austenworld, *withdrawing* from the idea that one drink isn't "quite sufficient" for happiness.

"The Proper Size"

Now for "some particulars." If Jane Austen were a barmaid, what would be her typical pour? Would she stint us like Mr. Woodhouse?—"what say you to *half* a glass of wine? A *small* half-glass . . . I do not think it could disagree with you." Hardly. Emma later returns and makes "all the amends in her power," topping everyone off with "full glasses of wine." But hang on, that's not as recklessly pour-happy as it sounds. Regency wine glasses came with built-in portion controls. They were notoriously tiny, holding just two ounces of wine (one-quarter cup).[31] That means even when Austen's ladies go loosey-goosey with "a supernumerary glass or two," they're still well under the safe benchmark for daily alcohol consumption (the equivalent of five ounces of wine). Most Americans drink dangerously past that limit in just their first glass, thanks to modern wine glasses now holding "normal" pours of seven to nine ounces. Studies have confirmed the obvious chain reaction: the bigger your wine glass, the more you pour, the more you ultimately drink,[32] a fact even Austen had to remind herself of. The "proper size" of alcoholic drinks is smaller than you might suspect: the new "wine glasses are much smaller than I expected," she wrote her sister in 1800, "but I suppose it is the proper size."

Summer Spruce Beer

Makes 1 cup of concentrated syrup

"Mr. Knightley had been telling him something about brewing spruce beer . . . and Mr. Elton's seeming resolved to learn to like it too."
—*Emma*

The piney flavor of Regency spruce beer can be replicated more easily today by substituting rosemary and lemon for the original spruce leaves. Added to sparkling mineral water, the fragrant syrup makes a refreshing alternative to modern soda.

INGREDIENTS

1 lemon

2 sprigs fresh rosemary (each sprig roughly 5 inches long)

1 cup water

1 cup sugar

¼ teaspoon ground ginger

Sparkling mineral water

1. Using a vegetable peeler, shave off long strips of zest from the entire lemon (avoiding the bitter white pith and saving the whole lemon to juice later). Put the lemon peel in a small saucepan with the rosemary and water. Bring the liquid to a full boil. Boil vigorously for 1 minute, then remove from the heat.

2. Add the sugar and ginger to the hot liquid, stirring to dissolve. Set aside until completely cool, leaving the rosemary and lemon peel to infuse the syrup.

3. When cool, remove and discard the rosemary and lemon peel. Juice the leftover lemon, adding about 3 tablespoons of fresh lemon juice to the syrup. Stir to combine.

4. Transfer the syrup to a pourable container of your choice. Refrigerate or use immediately, adding about 1 to 2 tablespoons of the concentrated syrup per cup of cool, sparkling mineral water. The syrup also adds a delightful zing to tea, either hot or iced.

"We are brewing spruce beer again . . . "
—Austen's letters

AUSTEN EATS:
MEAT

Advanced apologies to the eighteenth-century politically correct, but one can't properly begin a chapter on Regency meat attitudes without stooping to a little name calling. Boys will be boys, and naughty racial slurs have been hurled between the English and French (not exactly besties) since the Norman conquest. But it wasn't until the 1700s when the French came up with their most famous zinger. They started calling the English *les rosbifs*, "the roast beefs." I know, not a very war-rousing insult, but incredibly accurate. For centuries, the English were passionate meat eaters, enamored by their succulent joints of roast beef and anything else they could stick on a spit or stew in a pot—venison, pork, mutton, poultry, fish, sausage, the odd hare, should it present itself. Meat was the unquestioned king of the English table; the *rosbif* caricature was only a matter of time. Though, to be fair, the English started calling the French *frogs* (after their continental appetite for amphibians), so all's fair in love and war. Sort of. The English clearly felt they had scored one up on the rascally French. Eating meat wasn't a sign of national weakness, they thought, but one of their best cultural strengths, especially in matters of health. *Les rosbifs* became a backhanded compliment to happily embrace. And nobody was more sorry-not-sorry about her meat-eating values than Jane Austen.

"The Comforts of Cold Ham and Chicken"

Meat garners more attention in Jane's novels than any other food. If there's a luncheon with Lydia in *Pride and Prejudice*, the table will be "set out with such cold meat as an inn larder usually affords." If there's a picnic in *Emma*, the only foods referenced are "pigeon pies" and "cold lamb." Ditto the dinner party at the Weston's; there are other dishes on the table, of course, but only a "saddle of mutton" gets an honorable mention.

It's all part of Austen's sly class-ranking system: Jane's roundabout way of saying that most of her characters are living a "genteel" lifestyle. Since only the Regency rich and financially comfortable could afford regular meat in their diet, protein was the most prestigious food on anyone's table at the time. In Austenworld, protein equals prosperity.

Movie buffs will remember that meat is the last luxury food the once-wealthy Dashwoods reluctantly part with in the 1995 remake of *Sense and Sensibility*. "Surely you are not going to deny us beef?" says Mrs. Dashwood with a huff, evidently not enjoying her undignified spiral into poverty.[1] First evil Fanny, then creaky old cottage, now no beef!—life properly stinks at the moment. Yet not for the likes of Mr. Bingley in *Pride and Prejudice*. The first news of his return to Netherfield comes via his house-keeper, busy buying up lots of meat for his homecoming dinner—yet another clue that Bingley is living the high life on five thousand pounds a year. Charlotte Lucas isn't doing too shabby either. Recently married to the financially stable Mr. Collins, the only jab Lady Catherine can make about Charlotte's elevated style of living is that her "joints of meat were too large for her family." That's like somebody today finding fault with your Maserati because it's too large for your driveway.

Meat held such value at the time, it even winds up on the list of family possessions to be auctioned off when the Austens needed ready cash in 1801. Listed among their household furniture, feather beds, carpets, and pianoforte to be sold off is (I kid you not) one "side of bacon"—proudly positioned among the "Valuable Effects at Steventon Parsonage."[2] In *Emma*, a similar present of pork makes a penniless Miss Bates fall into raptures: "My dear Miss Woodhouse—I come quite over-powered. Such a beautiful hind-quarter of pork! You are too bountiful!"

This was a world that appreciated meat. One look at a Regency dinner table confirms it. The protein (beef, mutton, pork) was always placed in the symbolic center of the table; only then would smaller dishes of vegetables and starches orbit humbly around the meat. In *The Art of Cookery Made Plain and Easy*, one of the most popular cookbooks of the era, eighteenth-century housekeepers were instructed to fill up their tables with a variety of delicious dishes, but only if they are "suitable to your Meat"[3]—capital *M* very much intended.

The English had a right to be a little protein proud. Their beef, lamb, and pork were considered some of the finest in the world. With livestock grazing on rich pastures and meadowlands, English meat had an international reputation for succulence. "The English roasts are particularly remarkable," noted a European traveler in 1748. "All English meat, whether it is of ox, calf, sheep, or swine, has a fatness and delicious taste."[4] This beloved "fatness" of English meat was—Hold on. Time out. Beloved *fatness*? Ah, yes, I see how that could be a tad confusing. This calls for an emergency digression from meat to clear up Austen's smart relationship with fat. Time for a quick pit stop. Actually, let's be fun and call it a William Pitt Stop (for those unaware, William Pitt was Britain's prime minister throughout most of Jane's life). And yes, my version of "fun" is making irrelevant historical puns. So without further ado:

A William Pitt Stop

If you want to know how Austen felt about fat, turn to the end of *Pride and Prejudice*. Mrs. Bennet has just thrown a scrumptious dinner party for Darcy and Bingley, and everybody is raving about the roasted haunch of venison. "The venison was roasted to a turn—and everybody said they never saw so fat a haunch." Yes, the hit of the entire party is a juicy, generously fat-speckled piece of meat. Writing that scene in the late eighteenth century, Jane assumed her readers would relate, unabashedly applauding fat with the best and healthiest of Austenworld. It's how the vast majority of human history has always felt: fat was something to be enjoyed and guiltlessly appreciated. People relished the thought of living off "the fat of the land." They gloried in sermons with biblical promises that spoke of the Lord making "unto all people a feast of fat things . . . of fat things full of marrow." And when Charles Lamb penned his famously sensuous *A Dissertation Upon Roast Pig* in 1822, people immediately understood why he praised the crackling fat on roast pork, calling it positively "ambrosian," like pure "manna" from heaven.[5] Everybody knew fat was fabulous.

Austen certainly wouldn't understand our fear of it today: why we choose skinless, lean chicken breasts over nice plump thighs, egg whites over yolks, or a light salad dressing over a hearty splash of oil and vinegar. *"Tis a sad business,"* and one that robs us of one of the greatest gustatory pleasures since infancy (human breast milk is roughly 40 percent saturated fat).[6] It was one of the simplest aha lessons Julia Child had to relearn while cooking and eating in France, that "fat gives things flavor."[7] Yet many still believe that going "low-fat" is their dietary lot in life, that the historic heyday of enjoying fat is dead and gone. But Regency reality check: it ain't over 'til the fat venison sings.

First, to clear up the major and still lingering misconception—fat doesn't make you fat. Confusingly, the English language uses the same word for both the fat in our food and the flab on our bodies, but one has very little to do with the other. In fact, fat is the least likely food to actually make us gain weight. Unlike carbs and sugar, fat is the one macronutrient that doesn't trigger the release of insulin in our bodies.[8] Insulin, as previously discussed, is the biological switch that tells your cells to store excess sugar energy as body fat. Prolonged peaks of insulin (from frequent consumption of carbs and sugar) are what make us fat. Not fat itself.

The most staggering evidence came in the 1960s when researchers began studying the Maasai people of Kenya, some of the biggest fat lovers in the world. With a nomadic diet heavily reliant on meat and copious quantities of milk (three to five liters daily), Maasai men could easily consume more than 60 percent of their daily calories in the form of fat. And yet it didn't reflect on their bodies. Despite getting only "light" exercise from daily walking, the Maasai stayed remarkably svelte and slender, weighing about 50 percent less than their American counterparts. What's more, even with their high saturated-fat intake, the Maasai were heart healthy, with little to no occurrence of heart attacks among the tribe.[9] Which brings us to the second misconception— fat doesn't give you heart disease or bad cholesterol.

The idea that fat, especially saturated fat, blocks up our arteries has been one of the longest-running American myths since the 1950s, but was finally debunked in 2010. After looking at twenty-one studies involving more than 300,000 people, the highly respected *American Journal of Clinical Nutrition* found that "there is no significant evidence for concluding that dietary saturated fat is associated with an increased risk of CHD [coronary heart disease] or CVD [cardiovascular disease]."[10] This came on the heels of similar findings from the Women's Health Initiative—the largest study to date to look at the long-term effects of a low-fat diet. Following forty-nine thousand women for ten years, the study eventually concluded that cutting out fat didn't reduce the risk of heart disease, nor did it help the women lose weight.[11] So-called fat paradoxes have supported this for decades. Beginning with the French Paradox (when researchers first noticed that the French have much *lower* rates of heart disease than Americans despite eating *more* fat, butter, cream, and cheese), similar fat paradoxes have cropped up all over Europe. The sausage-loving Spaniards now have their Spanish Paradox and the cheese-loving Swiss their Alpine Paradox—all keeping healthy in spite of (or, perhaps, because of) their historic appreciation of fat. And since we're having ourselves a little paradox party, I'm inviting Austen. The Regency Paradox is just as fascinating. Not only were meat and fat highly esteemed in Austen's era, people saw them as inexorably linked with better health. Speaking of which, I hereby declare the William Pitt Stop officially over. Back to meat. Forthwith!

"She Ate Her Cold Meat; and Then She Was Well"

Being *les rosbifs* held a dual blessing for the English. The prestige and pleasure of eating meat ran parallel to the strong conviction that doing so kept them in hearty physical health (certainly healthier than the scrawny "frogs" across the channel). Since Tudor times, people like Thomas Elyot correlated the "health" of the English directly to the "Beef of England" which "bringeth strong nourishing."[12] In Austen's day, veritable hymns were sung to celebrate the connection. "Oh! the roast beef of Old England," went a favorite ditty composed by Henry Fielding. "It ennobled our brains and enriched our blood." The life-expectancy statistics seemed to agree. Around 1750, the English were living an average of ten years longer than the French.[13] Cue the update on the international scoreboard—Les Rosbifs: 1, Frogs: nil.

Got Gout?

Another meaty misunderstanding to clear up: red meat is often blamed for causing the iconic Regency affliction—gout. A painful form of arthritis, gout typically affects the feet, making sufferers feel as if they are, essentially, walking on their eyeballs (a gross and vivid description courtesy of eighteenth-century comedian Sydney Smith). There was indeed an unusually high incidence of gout in Austen's day—a "gout wave" as historians call it—which Jane often alludes to. But meat was likely the least cause. While meat consumption among the wealthy remained at traditional levels, wine consumption (especially wines from Portugal) spiked around the same time the "gout wave" occurred.[14] These eighteenth-century wines had infamously high levels of lead (from the lead in the wine casks to the *lead acetate*, "sugar of lead," used to sweeten the wines). And frequent lead poisoning can lead to, you guessed it, gout. It certainly explains why gout in the Regency era almost exclusively affected men (a fact reflected in Jane's novels). If you remember our "Drinks with Jane" chapter, it was usually only the men of the era that drank wine in abundance, thereby greatly increasing their risk of gout by lead poisoning. Another point for female *les rosbifs*!

We can hear Jane cheering from the bleachers in subtle but significant ways. In *Mansfield Park*, one of the first indicators that Fanny is in for a rough ride when staying with her poorer family in Portsmouth is a lack of meat. Arriving tired and hungry from the journey, she looks forward to a solid bit of protein to revive her. Her mother, however, only offers tea and toast, declaring: "we have no butcher" nearby and there isn't "time to dress a steak." Fanny endures this irregular meat pattern for three months and starts looking downright peaky because of it: "Her looks were . . . affected." "She had lost ground as to health since her being in Portsmouth." And yet the opposite occurs in *Persuasion*. Feeling unwell and listless for most of the morning, Mary finds her "cure" in a bit of protein. "She could soon sit upright . . . then, she ate her cold meat; and then she was well enough to propose a little walk." But how accurate is Austen's historic belief in meat? Caution: vegetarians might want to abandon ship now. We'll meet up again in the next chapter.

No . . . really . . . hop off—you're not going to like this.

Humans are genetically designed to thrive on meat. Almost every vitamin, mineral, and amino acid our bodies need to function properly is found in meat—it's nature's most complete multivitamin. The only essential nutrient *not* readily found in cooked meat is vitamin C (though even that's found in raw liver and fish roe). Meat is so nutritionally complete, with its natural combination of proteins and fats, humans can realistically live off nothing else, known as a ketogenic diet. All other nutritional combinations are inadequate for long-term survival: carbohydrates and vegetable proteins lack essential fats; carbohydrates and fat lack essential amino acids. Only meat holds the total package. Compare that to strict vegetarian and vegan diets, both requiring artificial supplements of vitamins (like B12) crucial to brain health and only found in meat.

Before the advent of modern supplements, people who ate more meat were essentially gulping down the historic equivalent of more vitamin pills. They were healthier, taller, and stronger. The most extreme example came in the early 1900s when the Icelandic anthropologist Vilhjalmur Stefansson spent a year living among the Inuit of the Canadian Arctic. The Inuit subsisted almost entirely off fatty meat (from caribou, salmon, eggs, and raw liver—vitamin C) and got very little exercise in the winter months. "They should have been in a wretched state," said Stefansson, "But, to the contrary, they seemed to me the healthiest people I had ever lived with."[15]

Obviously, Austen and her characters are not of the Arctic Inuit persuasion (heaven help Mr. Woodhouse if it snows more than a foot). They preferred their rounded English fare of vegetables, fruit, and a smattering of bread and other carbs, but meat unquestionably bulked out their diet. Following the advice in popular cookbooks like *The Art of Cookery Made Plain and Easy*, gentlefolk like Darcy and Bingley would have sat down to dinner with more than half of the table covered in meat dishes. Regency elegance still reigned—these weren't medieval moments for gnawing and belching into the nearest turkey leg (nobody in Austenworld eats more than a dainty "slice" of meat at a time). But nevertheless, interesting things happen when the majority of your calories come from meat.

Eating a slightly higher ratio of protein and fat (less of carbs and sugar) enables your pancreas to produce more of the hormone *glucagon*. Acting like insulin in reverse, glucagon signals your body to burn its own energy reserves (body fat) rather than rely on instant energy from carbs or sugar. Returning to healthier glucagon levels is the primary reason why people tend to lose excess body fat so quickly when they swap out carbs for meat. It's also one of the top secrets for how people like Austen effortlessly maintained their weight without ever technically "diet-ing" (i.e., starving themselves). There's a reason why the most approved snacks in Jane's novels usually involve meat. "Go and eat," says Emma, recommending "another slice of cold meat" to a hungry Frank Churchill in need of a quick snack. Protein and fat are the only foods that keep your body in fat-burning mode. Paradoxically, meat is the only true "fat-free" snack there is.

And while period dramas might make it look like there's an awful lot of meat on the tables of Austenworld, this was mostly a matter of show: another social cue that the wealthy could afford these vitamin-packed proteins in abundance. Regency tables, however, functioned more like elegant, variety-rich buffets; people weren't expected to eat everything in sight. Instead, the "habit and custom," wrote social observer John Ashton, is that people made "a judicious and careful selection from this little bazaar of good things"—winding up, perhaps, with little more than "a slice of turkey," "a sausage," and "a slice of tongue" on their plates.[16] Served one of these "magnificent" feasts at an inn in 1801, Austen jokes about the superabundance, saying that she and her companions "could not with the utmost exertion consume above the twentieth part of the beef." This is because all meat has a built-in satiety regu-lator. In other words, it's very difficult to eat large quan-tities of it. Since protein and fat are digested slowly, they fill you up quicker and satiate you longer than carbs and sugar. For instance, most people find it near impossible to eat a dozen eggs, but can easily polish off a typical bowl of pasta (about the same number of calories) and still feel hungry afterward. This appears to have been common sense in Austen's day. The most opulent Regency dinners always started with a first course of predominantly meat dishes. Then, only after the diners started to fill up on the meat would the starchier and sweeter dishes appear in the second and third courses.

Now to translate all of this into the reality of modern life, where three-course dinners are slightly harder to come by. Perhaps you've noticed I've avoided one term throughout this chapter with noticeable fear and trembling: that is, describing Austen as being on some sort of—cringe—"high-protein diet" program. (Hmm? Did you say *"shudderings of horror,"* Jane? Quite right). I avoided the high-protein label because it isn't technically true. Jane never forced herself to avoid bread or sweets, as we've already seen, and she certainly embraced the bounty of English produce with progressive zeal (as we'll see later). But for those who like things to be labeled nice and tidy, I think we can safely define Austen as happily living on a "meat-priority" diet. That is, when meat was on the table, she instinctually knew what to put her fork into first. Like the Bates in *Emma* and the cash-strapped Dashwoods in *Sense and Sensibility*, Jane didn't always have the luxury of living the full Regency meat life. But she prioritized it when it came. In 1805, when Jane received the Regency version of a "meat gift basket"—two plump and delicious pheasants from a generous friend—the meat naturally took precedence. "We shall live upon pheasants; no bad life!" she told her sister. More valuable and more nutritious, the choice was easy. Three centuries later, this meat-priority pattern is still the only sane protein "diet" for the real world. For instance, when you have a steak and potato, don't nix the potato, just eat more of the steak. When you're tackling a plate of meatballs and spaghetti, eat more meatballs than spaghetti. After all, when refreshments are served at Pemberley in *Pride and Prejudice*, there's cake and fruit to enjoy, but meat is proudly and conspicuously listed first: "[In came the] servants with cold meat, cake and a variety of all the finest fruits in season." *Les rosbifs* don't live on meat alone, they simply rank it above the rest. *Mais oui.*

William Pitt Stop: Part Deux

I'm afraid our first William Pitt Stop didn't cover the most fascinating and, perhaps, the most important aspect of Austen's relationship with fat: the omega balance. Like us, Jane's diet naturally included essential fatty acids omega-3s and omega-6s. They're "essential" because both are crucial to health. But balance is key. Historically, people eating traditional diets like Jane consumed far fewer omega-6s than we do today. This is cause for concern, since omega-6s (while helpful) are also biologically inflammatory. Unlike omega-3s that counteract damaging inflammation throughout the body, an overabundance of omega-6s in our diet can worsen it. Many health experts now see the highly lopsided omega ratio in modern Western diets—often as high as 15:1 (15 times more omega-6s than omega-3s)—as an obvious link in the current surge of inflammatory conditions from heart disease to cancer. In stark contrast, Austen, like most traditional eaters before the twentieth century, had an omega ratio in her diet of about 2:1 (only twice as many omega-6s as omega-3s)—a much healthier and more natural balance.[17] So how did she do it? Quite effortlessly, in fact, by sticking to historic food rules many of us have forgotten.

Field to Fork. The cows grazing in Austenworld's pastures aren't just bucolic, they're crucial to better health. When livestock are free to roam outside, eating their natural diet of grass and the occasional bug, their meat develops naturally higher levels of omega-3s (not to mention more vitamins, minerals, and antioxidants). What we would now call "grass-fed" beef has roughly the same amount of healthy omega-3s as omega-6s. Most modern beef, however, raised in a factory feedlot, has about seven times as many omega-6s as omega-3s—a consequence of the high-grain diet they're now fed, a highly inflammatory diet that ultimately passes on more omega-6s to us.[18] Though admittedly, I'm with you, traditionally raised grass-fed meat isn't cheap. But it does return the true value of meat to more accurate Regency levels. That "butcher meat" is expensive is a frequent observation in Jane's letters.

Eat Wild. Wild meat like fish and game were must-haves on Regency tables. In *Pride and Prejudice*, Mrs. Bennet launches into a tizzy when she can't get "a bit of fish" for her special dinner, while Sir John kindly fills the Dashwood's larder with "a present of game" in *Sense and Sensibility*. Both options prove excellent for keeping one's omega balance in check. Fish is a no-brainer (with its high omega-3 content in cold-water species), but game is also a healthy option. The benefit of eating more greens and grubs in the wild makes game another rich source of omega-3s.[19] During the "shooting season," Regency tables were replete with an incredible variety of game from partridge to pigeon. Though don't get your petticoats in a tangle—I'm not advising you to pick up a musket, traipse down to Longbourn, and "shoot as many [birds] as you please." Rather, just head to the supermarket. Most are now stocked with "exotic" game options: bison, goose, pheasant, and that perennial Regency favorite, venison.

Butter Up. To really get into the Regency omega groove, you'll have to rethink your relationship with vegetable oil. I'm not talking about olive oil, which has been around for thousands of years (and which frequently made its way into Regency salads), but industrial newcomers like canola oil, corn oil, soybean, safflower, and sunflower oil. These highly processed vegetable oils were only introduced into American diets in the 1920s; they have high amounts of omega-6s and are largely responsible for the omega imbalance in modern diets.[20] Yet they were totally absent from Austen's kitchen, and everyone else's kitchen in Europe and America from the nineteenth century backward. Instead, people almost entirely relied on animal fats to cook with—tallow, lard, suet, and, Austen's personal favorite, butter. Not only do these animal fats (from traditionally raised livestock) have a healthier omega balance, they are also more heat stable. Unlike modern vegetable oils that chemically oxidize when heated in the skillet (creating highly toxic compounds called *aldehydes* that can damage our cells), animal fats remain much more molecularly stable when heated.[21] Butter, of course, was the Regency standby. Rich in vitamin A and healthy fats from pasture-raised cows, you can get closest to the flavorful butter Austen would have eaten by sticking with grass-fed options (such as Kerrygold butter from Ireland, now widely available).

Mrs. Elton's Cold "Pigeon" Pie for Picnics

Serves 8

"It was now the middle of June, and the weather fine; and Mrs. Elton was growing impatient to name the day, and settle with Mr. Weston as to pigeon-pies and cold lamb."
—*Emma*

Seen in practically every Austen movie, hearty meat pies are still an English picnic tradition. Served cold like a rustic terrine, they're made with a "hot water crust," a pliable and sturdy pastry strong enough to hold a hefty quantity of meat. In this case, the original "pigeon" is swapped out for another Regency delicacy—turkey.

PIE FILLING

1 pound boneless turkey breast	2 tablespoons chopped sage
1 pound bacon	1½ teaspoons salt
1 pound pork sausage meat	4 tablespoons apricot preserves

CRUST

3½ cups all-purpose flour	1½ teaspoons salt
1 cup water	1 egg, beaten for brushing
¾ cup (6 ounces) natural lard (*not* hydrogenated)	Also needed: parchment paper and a 9-inch springform pan

1. For the filling: cut the turkey and bacon into small chunks. Transfer to a large bowl along with the sausage meat, sage, and salt. Using your hands, mix until well combined. Set aside.

2. For the crust: put the flour into a large heatproof bowl. In a saucepan combine the water, lard, and salt and heat on the stove until the lard melts and the water gently boils. Pour the hot liquid over the flour and stir with a wooden spoon until a solid dough forms. Cover the bowl with a damp dishcloth and leave until the dough is cool enough to handle. Preheat oven to 350°F.

3. When pleasantly warm, cut off ⅔ of the dough to roll out, leaving the rest under the cloth. For easy rolling, place dough between two sheets of parchment paper. Roll dough into a circle wide enough to cover the base and sides of a springform pan. Remove the top layer of parchment and, for easy transferring, roll up the dough within the bottom layer of parchment.

4. Unroll the dough over the springform pan (peeling off the parchment) and pushing down to cover the bottom and sides of the pan. The dough only needs to come up to the brim of the pan, so use any overhanging dough to patch together any holes or weak spots. Press the dough snugly into the sides and bottom of the pan.

5. Put half of the meat mixture into the pan, packing evenly down. Spread the apricot preserves over the meat. Pack the remaining meat mixture evenly over the apricot preserves. Brush the top edge of the dough with the beaten egg.

6. Using the parchment method, roll out the remaining dough to make a lid just wide enough to cover the top of the pan. Roll up the dough in the parchment and unroll over the top of the meat mixture (the dough will "sit" in the pan slightly). Press around the edges to seal dough together.

7. Cut off any overhanging dough. Crimp the edges of the dough to make a pretty ripple effect. Cut a small, nickel-sized hole in the center of the pie to let steam escape. Brush only the top of the dough with the egg (not the crimped edge: that will get browned enough in the oven).

8. Put the pan on a baking sheet and bake for 1 hour and 30 minutes. The crust should be a rich golden brown. Let the pie cool slightly before covering with foil and chilling in the refrigerator overnight. Serve cold (with mustard and pickles) at your next picnic.

"Cold provisions were to be taken, open carriages only to be employed, and everything conducted in the usual style of a complete party of pleasure."
—*Sense and Sensibility*

"Yesterday was a busy day with me,
or at least with my feet and stockings."
—*Austen's Letters*

5

WALK LIKE AN ELIZABETH: EXERCISE IN AUSTENWORLD

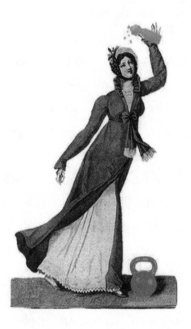

It's difficult to imagine Jane using the word *exercise* at all. Surely her innocent mind never knew the cruel tortures that word now encapsulates. The sweat and pain when we do it, the guilt and shame when we don't—only to repeat again tomorrow (or next New Year's for those completely pummeled by the experience). Is there any ruder reminder that we're *not* living in a Jane Austen novel?

And yet, Jane *does* use the word *exercise*, uses it quite a lot, as a matter of fact. Uses it, loves it, wraps a Regency ribbon around it and gifts it to her heroines like a life-changing lottery ticket—"Is there a felicity in the world . . . superior to this?"—and all without the slightest trace of sadism. There are over a hundred reminders to exercise in Jane's novels, and not one of them is laced with "guilt and misery," or more sweat than Regency elegance would allow. No, the tale of exercising in Austenworld is "a different story" altogether.

For one, exercise in Jane's novels is *only* viewed as something fun and enjoyable, "the pure genuine pleasure of the exercise," she calls it. Austen heroines exercise because they *want* to, not because they *have* to. It's a legitimate treat. Lizzie likes to "indulge herself in . . . exercise." Catherine "gave herself up to all the enjoyment of . . . exercise." And Anne experiences genuine "pleasure . . . from the exercise." Words like "comfortable," "delightful," and even "snug" define their daily workouts, with nobody getting too strenuous or pushing their bodies to any level of physical pain. "A face glowing with the warmth of exercise" is about the most intense aftereffect you're likely to get while exercising in Austenworld.

Anyone who's been to a gym in the last decade will find all of this fantastically (even amusingly) odd. The ground rules are so different there, condensed into something cheery like: no workout is *really* effective unless it ends with you flailed on the floor in breathless agony.

More hardcore gyms put up helpful posters, just in case us namby-pamby weaklings forget it. "Crawling is acceptable, falling is acceptable, puking is acceptable, crying is acceptable, blood is acceptable, pain is acceptable. Quitting is not!"[1] Austen would only roll her eyes and tell us to lighten up. Lizzie's eyes are only ever "brightened by . . . exercise," never teared by it.

Because it turns out, Jane's advice to keep exercise as light, pleasurable, and easy as possible isn't a sign of weakness at all, but of brilliant scientific sense. Humans have a built-in reflex to avoid discomfort whenever we can. Embracing the modern "no pain, no gain" compulsion to exercise might sound powerful and plucky, but your brain and biology will constantly rail against it, and usually win. Austen figured this out in *Mansfield Park*: "Nothing ever fatigues me, but doing what I do not like." It's the main reason why strict exercise regimens are so difficult to maintain, why New Year's fitness resolutions end by February, and why gyms have some of the biggest dropout rates on the planet. An infinitesimally few of us actually like what exercise has become. Our biggest problem: we've gotten far beyond what Austen knew and loved about truly effective exercising in the first place.

"The Felicities of Rapid Motion"

Jane's novels are some of the first books to embrace what we would now call "intuitive exercise"—the belief that simply being "in motion" feels good and is good for our bodies (far better than trying to endlessly force them beyond their biological comfort zone). A more accurate word to encapsulate Austen's broader exercise philosophy would be *motion-cise* (alas, if only it didn't sound like a 1980s step-aerobics class). Because the characters with the simple drive to move more, to enjoy the "felicities of rapid motion," are the healthiest, fittest, happiest people in Austenworld.

"I am not born to sit still and do nothing," says the vivacious Mary Crawford in *Mansfield Park*, spurning all attempts to keep her down. "After sitting a little while, Miss Crawford was up again," saying, "I must move . . . resting fatigues me." In *Northanger Abbey*, all other girls are "insipid" compared to Catherine Morland, who finds that "nothing but motion was voluntary" to her. "Catherine . . . was not naturally sedentary" and "it seemed as if she would even walk about the house rather than remain fixed for any time in the parlour." The same love for frequent movement is shared by Emma, Elinor, Marianne, and Lizzie—whose fondness for being frequently up and about comes across as "almost wild" to the sedentary, needle-pointing Bingley sisters.

"I Must Move"

It's worth noting how revolutionary these energetic female characters were for the time. Like most women of the era, Jane grew up in a world that defined femininity in far less animated terms.

To then contemporary male thinkers like Edmund Burke, female beauty "always carries with it an idea of weakness . . . Women are very sensible of this: for which reason they learn to lisp, to totter in their walk, to counterfeit weakness, and even sickness."[2] This peeved proto-feminist Mary Wollstonecraft, who labeled such talk "ridiculous jargon."[3] And it angered Austen too. "Do not consider me now as an elegant female . . . but as a rational creature," says Lizzie to Mr. Collins, proving her true feminine strength with a flaunting "quick step" out of the room.

As for the more stationary bodies of Austenworld, Jane is equally clear about the consequences. "Ill health" and "a great deal of indolence" define Lady Bertram in *Mansfield Park*, her bum permanently plastered to the sofa throughout the novel. Another perpetual sitter, Mr. Woodhouse in *Emma*, looks and feels "a much older man" than he really is. "Without activity . . . of body," a simple half-mile stroll is beyond his comprehension. It is "such a distance," he mutters weakly, "I could not walk half so far." Then there's *Persuasion*, where we first meet Mary Musgrove "lying on the faded sofa," and soon pick up on Austen's hint that Mary's frequent illnesses are a direct result of her "not being supposed a good walker."

This was common knowledge circa 1800. Georgian doctors viewed the body as a sort of machine (the *machina carnis*, they called it) that needs regular movement to work properly.[4] "There must be frequent motions," said Joseph Addison in 1711, or the "engine" of the body is liable to rust up.[5] It's why Austen characters, people like Frank Churchill in *Emma*—who sit "still when he ought to move"—are always playing a risky game with their health.

It's fascinating to witness how modern science has recently returned to that core belief. The very un-Regency phenomenon of seeing exercise as only that sweaty thing you do between this-and-that o'clock is entirely wrong. Moving more *throughout* the day is now regarded as markedly healthier than spending an exhausting hour at the gym after a full day of sitting. Your body is indeed a sort of *machina carnis*, a biological engine that runs best when you move it more frequently (not necessarily more vigorously)—a fact first "rediscovered" in 1953 when scientists in Britain observed that workers who stood or moved more throughout the day (i.e., train conductors on their feet collecting fares, postmen on their bikes delivering letters) had less coronary heart disease than workers with more sedentary jobs (bus drivers, office workers).[6] Sitting for a prolonged period of time throughout the day (à la Lady Bertram) effectively shuts your body engine down: muscles stop firing, blood stops circulating properly, and the mechanisms that regulate healthy blood sugar and cholesterol levels deteriorate—all dramatically increasing your risk of obesity, heart disease, and diabetes.[7]

"Sitting is the new smoking," say umpteen-thousand articles published every year, no doubt a happy vindication for Mrs. Norris in *Mansfield Park*. "Idling away all" your time "upon a sofa" is "a very foolish trick." But those articles are a bore, Mrs. Norris is a twit, and Austen, you'll remember, never liked to "dwell on guilt and misery." So let's quickly turn to her antidote for all of this "idleness and folly"—the best ways to get moving with the best bodies of Austenworld. And it begins with nothing "beyond a walk."

"I Walk: I Prefer Walking"

I won't beat around the shrubbery. *Everything* happens on a walk in Jane's novels: Darcy proposes to Elizabeth on a walk; Marianne meets Willoughby on a walk; Lucy Steele drops the I'm-engaged-to-Edward bomb on a walk; Harriet is *nearly* attacked by gypsies on a walk (lives to tell the tale); Anne Elliot and Captain Wentworth hook up again on a walk.

Yet none of this feels remotely clichéd or unconvincing, as if Jane merely ran out of convenient plot settings. On the contrary, her novels' most important walks usually fade seamlessly into the fabric of ordinary life for her characters. These people are walking *all the time* anyway. Just how much is quite impressive:

🏋 The Bennet girls in *Pride and Prejudice* walk six to eight miles every week, just by going back and forth from their home (at Longbourn) to the nearby village of Meryton: "The village of Longbourn was only one mile from Meryton; a most convenient distance for the young ladies, who were usually tempted thither three or four times a week."

149

🔔 The Dashwoods in *Sense and Sensibility* often "walked up from the cottage" to Sir John's residence at Barton Park—"a half mile" walk each way. Marianne is also on one of her usual walks, "about a mile and a half from the cottage" when she first sees Willoughby's house at Allenham.

🔔 The characters of *Persuasion* rack in some serious pedometer readings. Anne finds it "most natural" to make "a daily walk to Lady Russell's" house—half a mile each way. The same feeling is shared by the Musgrove clan. Though Uppercross Cottage and the Great House are "a quarter of a mile" apart, "the two families were so continually meeting, so much in the habit of running in and out of each other's house at all hours."

All of this "running in and out" quickly added up. It wasn't unusual for a Regency person, going visiting or walking to nearby villages, to easily rake in about seven miles in one day[8] (in addition to milling about around their house). Elizabeth Bennet, therefore, finds nothing very taxing in making the three-mile walk to Netherfield to visit Jane. "I do not wish to avoid the walk. The distance is nothing when one has a motive; only three miles, I shall be back by dinner." So off she trots: "crossing field after field at a quick pace, jumping over stiles and springing over puddles with impatient activity." Even the spiteful Bingley sisters concede that Lizzie is, if nothing else, "an excellent walker." She can easily walk along country lanes "for two hours" while reading Darcy's letter, and desperately wants to walk "round the whole park" of the Pemberley estate (a *mere* ten miles), but stops short because her aunt, "who was not a great walker, could go no farther." Even her marriage proposal isn't complete without a long walk with Darcy lasting "several miles." Small wonder, considering her creator was such a passionate walker too. Austen proudly styled herself as one of the "desperate walkers" of the world, "walking about and enjoying the air" whenever she could. One energetic day in 1805 brought these Lizzie-like tidings from Jane's correspondence: "Yesterday was a busy day with me, or at least with my feet and my stockings; I was walking almost all day long; I went to Sidney Gardens soon after one, and did not return till four, and after dinner I walked to Weston" (a mile and a half away).[9]

Austen naturally walked like an Elizabeth. Few of us can say the same today.

Actually, we're walking more like the Elizabeth on the modern movie posters of *Pride and Prejudice* (2005)—look to the bottom and you'll find a tiny Keira Knightley confined to the walking distance of a typical parking lot. That's basically the extent of our "walks" today: the distance between our cars and office, cars and supermarket, cars and home—giving the average American less than an hour of cumulative walking time per day.[10] And giving the rest of the world an endlessly amusing anecdote to tell their friends back home: "Yeah, I've seen it! They *do* get in their cars just to drive across the parking lot. Ha, ha.

Bloody Americans!" Somewhat old news to Austen, however, who's seen it all before.

Regency England was in a bit of a movement crisis too. Better roads and comfier carriages meant walking was now an *option* for more people than ever before. As one eighteenth-century doctor put it, the English gentry could now afford to be among "the lazy, the luxurious, and the inactive."[11] All over the country, the rich were being shuffled along in "sedan chairs." A sort of Regency people-mover on poles (carried by two miserable servants), sedan chairs could zip you from one house to the next, dropping you off in the front parlor if it struck your fancy. Across the continental pond the mood was basically the same. A French tourist visiting America in 1798 went away with one cultural impression: "Americans are in the habit of never walking, if they can ride."[12] Sound familiar? I'd call it a perfect reflection of modern life (if you compress "carriage" down to car), making Austen's intuitive "inclination to walk" so keenly appropriate today.

"I Would Rather Have Walked"

Regency carriages might have been comfier, but they still took a considerable time to "rev up" (servants had to be summoned, horses had to be harnessed). It was usually quicker to just walk. Especially when the destination was considered "a most convenient distance"—defined in Jane's novels as anything at or below one mile. Meryton's village shops are a mile away from the Bennet home; Mrs. Weston moves the "very easy distance" of a half-mile walk from Emma's place; and no self-respecting Austenite would dream of calling for the carriage for "such a little way." Although if walking less than a mile to visit a friend or pop into a shop doesn't seem so convenient nowadays, you might need to recalibrate your distance scale to Regency standards. Start on the easier end of Austen's walkable-distance rule. In *Sense and Sensibility*, Mrs. Dashwood defines her ideal "distance of a walk" as the quarter-mile stroll between her cottage and Barton Park—the same quarter-mile distance separating the two Musgrove houses in *Persuasion*. So think like a Regency walker. If the places you normally go (parks, stores, restaurants) are within a quarter-mile distance from you, consider walking to them instead. And never, ever repeat "that dreadful habit" of getting into your car to only drive across a parking lot. *"It is a compliment which I never pay to any place if I can avoid it."*

Only requiring a pair of "impatient feet," Jane knew that walking was (and still is) the easiest, cheapest, safest, most natural form of exercise we have. Done anytime, anywhere, without the drag of driving to a gym, walking has the lowest "dropout" rate of any other physical activity, according to the American Heart Association.[13] Jane's novels repeatedly bear out that fact.

Characters who rely on other forms of exercise don't move nearly as much as organic walkers like Lizzie. In *Mansfield Park*, Fanny relies solely on horseback riding as her only "means of exercise" (the Regency equivalent of relying solely on the gym) and is constantly being prevented from exercising at all. One excuse after another pops up and somebody (ahem, Mary Crawford) is *always* using the equipment she wants. Consequently, Fanny's overall physical-fitness level is embarrassingly low. A mere half-mile walk and she's "knocked up" with exhaustion for the day. Not exactly the quickest heroine in the Park, Fanny apparently hasn't figured out what everyone else in Austenworld intuitively knows: "when she does not ride, she ought to walk."

Historically, the simple act of walking has kept more people fit, healthy, and trim than any exercise gadget invented in the last century. And interestingly, those who have stuck closest to a Regency walking lifestyle—the Amish, for instance—have some of the leanest bodies on earth. A pedometer study in 2004 found that in one Canadian Amish community, the women walked an average of fourteen thousand steps a day (about seven miles, a familiar figure to any active Austenite). And despite a diet rich in hearty farm fare—meat, butter, potatoes, bread— the prevalence of obesity within the community was rare. Only 9 percent of the women were obese, compared to an obesity rate of 30 percent among Americans.[14] As Darcy reminds us, our "figures appear to the greatest advantage in walking." Being an "excellent walker" certainly works out for Lizzie in the physical department. Her three-mile walk to Netherfield (attractively glowing with "the brilliance exercise had given to her") practically seals her fate as the future mistress of Pemberley.

In Austenworld, a life can quickly change on a walk because "walk" and "life" were two concepts closely connected for Jane. One of the last orders she gives her characters in *Persuasion* is the order to walk more: "to walk for her life." Today, that order is as literal as ever. And experiencing the life-changing magic of a "daily walk" starts by remembering her ground rules:

1. "The Whole Walk Was Delightful . . . "

The first rule of Austen Walk Club: there are no rules in Austen Walk Club. In *Northanger Abbey*, Catherine and Henry are at their happiest when walking is viewed as purely a "voluntary" activity: "walking where they liked and when they liked, their hours, pleasures, and fatigues, at their own command." Turns out, even laboratory mice feel the same, naturally hopping on and off running wheels at their own enjoyable pace. But force them to exercise and the stress involved can easily outweigh the benefits.[15] How much Austen grasped this is evident by how conspicuously she kept herself from issuing any stringent walking guidelines. You'll find an incredible diversity of walkers and walking options in her novels—fast walkers, slow walkers, morning walks, afternoon walks, evening walks, even moonlit walks—all bound by nothing more than the sheer "exquisite enjoyment" of the activity. How you think about walking matters. A fascinating study in 2014 confirmed that people who *thought* they were walking "for exercise" rather than simply walking for pleasure were much more likely to reward themselves with unhealthy food choices for completing the activity.[16] In Austenworld, walking *itself* is the feel-good reward.

2. "There Is Nothing So Refreshing as a Walk"

If Austen characters have one biological motive for walking more, it's literally in their minds. Walking appears to magically boost and balance their mental health. Jane makes countless references to moods, feelings, and "spirits" being cheered and "freshened up" by walking. It's one of her most reliable physiological litmus tests—Austen characters who walk more are measurably happier than those who don't. People who are "not in the habit of walking" much, like Mrs. Bennet, tend to have "gloomy thoughts," while others, like Lizzie, naturally turn to walking to alleviate stress and anxiety: "she walked up and down the room . . . to compose herself." It's Austen's acknowledgement of an ancient belief—the concept that walking can effectively "clear your head"—and one dating back to Greek philosophy (*solvitur ambulando*, "it is solved by walking," went the classical motto). But it wasn't until 1999 that this belief was scientifically confirmed. A landmark study by Duke

University found that quick walking (for thirty minutes, three times a week) was just as effective as antidepressants in relieving the symptoms of major depression—and, over the long term, even more effective than medication.[17] An almost identical claim is made by Jane Fairfax in *Emma*—"quick walking will refresh me . . . we all know at times what it is to be wearied in spirits." Moreover, the same Duke University study discovered that walking tends to boost people's confidence, giving them heightened feelings of self-regard. Is it any coincidence that the most iconic walker in Austenworld (Lizzie Bennet) is also the most iconically self-confident? "Obstinate, headstrong girl!" says Lady Catherine, the best backhanded compliment in the book.

3. "I Should Be Glad to Take a Turn"

While a "nice long walk" is a lovely treat in Austenworld, even Regency schedules didn't always allow for them every day. Heck, the accomplished woman has to improve "her mind by extensive reading" sometime! So when compelled to sit for long periods, Austenites rely on a handy trick to keep them frequently on their feet—*taking a turn*. I'll try to explain this without sounding hopelessly disconnected from modern reality. Taking a turn is merely rising from your chair and pacing around whatever space is at your disposal. Here's Caroline Bingley's explanation in *Pride and Prejudice*: "let me persuade you to follow my example, and take a turn about the room. —I assure you it is very refreshing after sitting so long in one attitude." To quickly vindicate both of us, taking frequent "turns" throughout the day has indeed been shown to refresh you on a biological level. Even just two minutes of light walking (for every twenty minutes of sitting) significantly reduces both blood sugar and insulin levels[18]—two things always dangerously out of whack when sitting for prolonged periods. Remembering the Regency wisdom of "taking a turn" is especially crucial for desk workers (like me). So three cheers to anyone clever enough to invent the app we've all been waiting for: one that periodically pings on our desks with Caroline's sassy voice: "Let me persuade you to take another turn about the room . . . "

4. "The Whole Country . . . Abounded in Beautiful Walks"

It's unanimous. Austen characters prefer exercising outside: whether that's "scampering about the country," walking along garden paths, or climbing the hilly "downs, rejoicing in their own penetration at every glimpse of blue sky." And that's *not* because Jane didn't have access to a gym. The Regency era, in fact, had its fair share of indoor exercise options. There was the "chamber horse," for one—a bouncy exercise chair that hilariously mimicked the up-and-down motion of horseback riding (though I dare say most of our modern fitness gadgets will be equally hilarious in two hundred years). Then there was the Regency version of the treadmill—walking in endless circles in indoor spaces like the pump room at Bath. Catherine experiences its mind-numbing dullness in *Northanger Abbey*: "Every morning . . . they paraded up and down [the pump room] for an hour, looking at everybody and speaking to no one"—the most tedious "exercise" in Jane's novels. For good reason. Countless studies have confirmed Austen's intuition that "fatigues within doors . . . are worse." People who swap out the gym for the great outdoors consistently find exercising more pleasurable, more invigorating, and less tiring than when performing the same exercise indoors.[19] The TVs, air-conditioning, and giant mirrors of indoor gyms simply can't compete with the residual health benefits of getting outside, "where the opening of the trees gave the eye power to wonder," where the nuance effects of natural light and fresh air act like the ultimate energy drink—something of deep significance to Jane, which we'll explore in the upcoming chapter, "A Taste for Nature."

"Run Mad as Often as You Choose, but Do Not Faint"

Now to tackle the running question: Did Jane ever run? Did she approve of it? Surprisingly, there's quite a lot of "running about" in her novels, and all of it generally positive. For Marianne, the "one consolation" of having to hurry home during a rainstorm is the enjoyment "of running with all possible speed down the steep side of the hill which immediately led to their garden gate." In *Pride and Prejudice*, Lizzie beats her sister in a running match through the house and garden because Lizzie enjoyed "the habit of running" more frequently than Jane. But all of this running comes in sporadic bursts. Nobody runs (i.e., jogs) for prolonged periods of time in Austenworld. Running for too long, over unnaturally long distances, would have defied Austen's guiding health principle: "moderation in all things." Historically speaking, long-distance running has always been regarded as a rather dubious form of exercise. If you remember your Greek history, the first marathon runner of the ancient world collapsed dead at the finish line. As Austen would say, "there are very few of us who have heart enough" for it. Carried on for too long, the sheer heart-pumping intensity of running can dangerously enlarge, harden, and overstretch the heart muscle itself. Endurance runners are infamously prone to heart damage,[20] and some of the most famous have suffered heart attacks while still young. Moderation, therefore, should keep you, as it kept Jane, from ever "running into any excess." Walk mostly and only run occasionally, remembering that being "absolutely out of breath from haste" is not a prolonged sensation in Austenworld.

We'll finish our walk with Jane by not forgetting to take a "refreshing" rest from time to time. Like the intuitive exercisers they are, Austen characters listen to their bodies, know when they need a break, and never pressure themselves to "power through." Enjoying a guiltless rest was certainly part of Jane's broader exercise philosophy. "[I am] quite equal to walking about and enjoying the air, and by sitting down and resting a good while between my walks, I get exercise enough." Hence her fictional walks are always conveniently dotted with comfy benches—"A few steps farther brought them" to "a comfortable-sized bench, on which they all sat down." For all of us, these natural rest periods are crucial for keeping exercise pleasurable and in its proper place in our lives. Hippocrates, the world's first celebrity doctor, was saying it two thousand years ago: "The right amount of . . . exercise, not too much, not too little is the safest way to health."[21] Mary Bennet in *Pride and Prejudice* would only sniff and adjust her spectacles with an I-could-have-told-you-that expression. "Exertion" she kindly reminds us, "should always be in proportion to what is required."

Speaking of which, even resting has its hidden health secrets in Austenworld: a place where you can legitimately "exercise" without ever moving a delicate ankle. It starts by rethinking how you sit and stand.

"The Posture Is Thought Good for Me"

When the cast of *Sense and Sensibility* (1995) began preproduction training for their onscreen roles, one of their first lessons was learning the correct art of Regency posture. As Emma Thompson records in *The Sense and Sensibility Screenplay and Diaries*, the film's movement coach (Jane Gibson) had to teach the actors how to stand and sit like proper Austenites, offering this helpful historic reminder: It's 1811, "God is in his heaven, the monarch on his throne, and the pelvis firmly beneath the ribcage." Emma Thompson goes on to quip, "Apparently rock and roll liberated the pelvis and it hasn't been the same since."[22]

Most of us don't even notice how far we've fallen, or slumped, from Regency posture rules. But walk around any public space, then go watch the actors in *Sense and Sensibility* (especially the women) and the differences will be shocking. Forget liberated pelvises, we've liberated *everything*. Bellies, chests, shoulders, spines, necks all hang limp and loose, often hunched in a near permanent C-pattern in front of the closest screen. To Austen, it would look like we've all unanimously adopted what she called, "the posture of reclining weakness," a body-slouch Jane would have only associated with the sick, bedridden, or elderly. Because in Regency England, few things offered a stronger visual cue to someone's health and vitality than the simple fact that "she stood firm."

The attractiveness of good posture was deeply ingrained in the Regency mind. Enamored by the aesthetic fashions, art, and architecture of ancient Greece and Rome, Austen and her contemporaries loved all that was long and tall and firmly poised. "I admire" what is "tall, straight, and flourishing," says Edward Ferrars. Standing solidly upright (as straight as a Grecian pillar, as it were) was everyone's ideal of physical beauty and elegant strength. Francois Nivelon stressed the importance of striking this "graceful attitude" in his widely read posture manual, *The Rudiments of Genteel Behavior*: of always keeping the head "erect," the shoulders "drawn back," and the whole body serenely "firm."[23]

Anyone who has tried to maintain this "graceful attitude" for any extended length of time knows how physically challenging it is. After posture lessons on the set of *Sense and Sensibility*, Emma Thompson realized just how physically strong Austen women were underneath those delicate muslin gowns. She writes about the hidden "muscularity of their physique, the strength beneath the ease of movement."[24] Basically, Austenites get serious back and ab workouts even when standing or sitting still.

This explains why correct posture (maintained throughout the day) was deemed a legitimate exercise in Austen's day. The sheer strength involved in standing "with an air of decided fashion" was considerable. Walking tall and graceful wherever you went, as Caroline Bingley reminds us in *Pride and Prejudice*, was one of the physical "accomplishments" of Regency life. "No one can be really be esteemed accomplished who does not . . . possess a certain something in her air and manner of walking." And that applied to sitting too.

Regency gentlefolk rarely slouched back or reclined in a chair. Striking a straight figure while sitting was just as important as doing so while standing, a cultural rule reflected in practically every Austen movie to date: the backs of chairs and the backs of human bodies are perpetually kept asunder. Austen's nephew recalled this social rule in his memoir: "There were no deep easy-chairs, nor other appliances for lounging; for . . . to lean back, was a luxury permitted only to old persons or invalids."[25] Away from home was no different. While riding in carriages, healthy travelers always strived to maintain good posture—quite the physical feat considering the bumpiness of Regency roads. For Catherine in *Northanger Abbey*, a jostling joy ride in John Thorpe's gig along country roads means "exercise of the most invigorating kind." The next time you find yourself in an off-road vehicle on unpaved roads, try keeping your own back and core muscles straight, and you'll see what Catherine means—why good posture is one of the smartest Regency "exercises" we should all get back to embracing.

"She Is a Standing Lesson of How to Be Happy"

Putting aside the lamentable fact that I'm no Jane Gibson (Hollywood posture-coach extraordinaire) and we're not on the set of *Sense and Sensibility* (alas!), I'll try my best to make it up to you. Here's a quick reminder on what "correct posture" meant to Jane and what it still means for us today:

🏋 Think "tall, straight, and flourishing" whenever you stand, sit, or walk.

🏋 Keep your chin parallel to the floor and your neck even with your shoulders.

🏋 Straighten your back, but avoid over-arching the spine or puffing out your chest too far. Only Regency wenches thrust out their bosoms like that!

🏋 Tighten your abs to keep your hips and pelvis, as Jane Gibson instructed, "firmly beneath the ribcage."

Put it all together and you'll be doing the Regency hokey pokey to better health in no time. Surprisingly, most people tend to experience almost instantaneous feelings of well-being whenever they stand or sit up straight. Your lungs fill up with more oxygen, your blood circulates more freely, and your muscles and joints instantly reward you for the much-needed stretch. What's more, science continues to discover that good posture sends out powerful and primal body signals, not only making us *look* healthier, smarter, stronger, and happier, but making us *feel* that way too. Experiments have shown that people who adopt better posture are less stressed, more positive, have better energy, and feel more confident than people who slouch.[26]

Jane's novels offer a litany of support for this. Whereas Lady Bertram in *Mansfield Park* is made self-evidently "stupid" by slouching every day on a sofa ("I cannot think," "I cannot work," "I feel so very stupid"), Austen's

165

most physically "upright" characters always have the first dibs on health and happiness—Mrs. Croft, most memorably. *Persuasion*'s patron saint of good posture, she reminds us that you don't have to be the tallest, slimmest, or most beautiful person in Austenworld to be "a most attractive picture of happiness." Good posture and a little "uprightness" goes a long way: "Mrs. Croft, though neither tall nor fat, had a squareness, uprightness, and vigour of form, which gave importance to her person."

Other Exercises in Austenworld

Dance: Nothing epitomizes Austen's knack for mixing exercise with pleasure than "the whirl of a ballroom." Dancing is called a "sport" in her novels, something her characters can play at for hours. Willoughby dances "from eight o'clock to four [a.m.], without once sitting down." Austen loved a good bop too. "There were twenty dances" at a local ball in 1798, "and I danced them all, and without any fatigue." As Sir Lucas points out in *Pride and Prejudice*: "There is nothing like dancing." One of the most natural cardio workouts, the urge to move along to music is imprinted on our DNA. Five-month-old babies automatically shake their bodies in response to rhythm, and every culture marks the happiest life moments through dance.[27] Of course, nobody *needs* to exercise by dancing. "It may be possible to do without dancing entirely," says Austen, "but when a beginning is made—when the felicities of rapid motion have once been, though slightly, felt—it must be a very heavy set that does not ask for more."

    Garden: Charlotte may have a *teensy* double motive in keeping Mr. Collins in the garden and as far away from her as physically possible: "Charlotte talked of the healthfulness of the exercise, and owned she encouraged it as much as possible." But others of the era had deep beliefs in its benefits. Since 1670, the English were advised to spend "spare time in the garden, either digging, setting out, or weeding," for "there is no better way to preserve your health."[28] Jane's mother (who lived to eighty-eight) gardened throughout her long life, once composing a few verses about the exercise: "My flesh is much warmer / my blood freer flows / When I work in the garden with rakes and with hoes."[29] Not only a legitimate workout for our bodies (spending thirty minutes planting a flower bed is the metabolic equivalent of a game of basketball lasting the same time), our brains reap benefits too. Pottering about in a garden (or just walking through one) reduces stress, lowers blood pressure, and refreshes us on a deep mental level.[30] For Jane, the best rooms for writing always opened "upon the garden. [Where] I go refresh myself every now and then, and then come back to Solitary Coolness."

Bathe: "A little sea-bathing would set me up forever," says Mrs. Bennet, referencing the most fascinating exercise of the era. On the surface, there doesn't seem to have been much to it. People went to the seaside (usually in winter), spent a minute or so "dipping" in the frigid ocean, then called it a day. More like bobbing in cold water than actual swimming, yet people swore by its health benefits. And this was exercise?! Interestingly, yes. Your body's biggest calorie-burning feature is keeping you warm (at an average 98.6 degrees), a huge energy-expending process called thermoregulation. And because your body is always trying to maintain that temperature, exposing it to anything cold (especially cold water) kicks thermoregulation into high gear, burning large amounts of calories and body fat to keep your innards warm. The ancient Romans knew it: that the best way to work up an appetite was a quick plunge into the *frigidarium*—a large cold bath. Health-conscious Russians and Scandinavians also swear by the exhilarating exercise of getting cold, requisitely jumping into cold lakes or rolling in snow after sauna treatments. And you can power up your own thermoregulator by spending more time in water (showers, baths, or swimming pools) colder than your body temperature. Braver souls who turn the tap colder will experience the same invigorating body effects Jane experienced on a sea-bathing trip in September of 1804: "I continue quite well; in proof of which I have bathed again this morning."

AUSTEN EATS:
CARBS

No, it's not your imagination. These chapters *have* been getting longer the more we progress. Though I like to think this ever-so-slight and very respectable chapter plumping hasn't been nearly as jarring as, say, finishing *Northanger Abbey* (239 pages) only to be pummeled by *Mansfield Park* (439 pages). By the way, remind me to ask Jane "what gives?" once we all get to Regency heaven one day. The woman has some serious explaining to do about *Mansfield Park* . . .

> Me: What's that, Jane?
> Jane: *I believe you "have gone quite distracted." Serious "material digression of thought" alert.*
> Me: Oh, right. Back to carbs.

I promise this will be a relatively short and snippy chapter. Austen has very little to say about carbs. In fact, Austen is so carb cautious throughout her novels, it's easy to assume that she was some sort of proto-champion of the Atkins or South Beach diet, boldly promoting a low-carb lifestyle two centuries before it was fashionable. But the main reason Jane is so silent about carbs, why they garner such little attention in her stories is, I am proud to say, much more entertaining than that. It all boils down to shameless Regency snootiness.

Whereas we might feel very chic sashaying up to the grocery checkout line with an expensive bag of whole-grain, hand-picked quinoa from darkest Peru, people in Regency England wouldn't be at all impressed. For them, most starchy foods were decidedly common and cheap. Belly filling and inexpensive throughout most of human history, carb-dense foods like beans, barley, dried peas, and oats had long been linked with the English peasantry. The poor souls who pulled ploughs and furrowed pastures all day long, the people Miss Steele would call "dirty and nasty," might have no choice but to settle down to a dense, cheap, and satisfying pot of pease porridge (some like it hot, some like it cold), but the rich didn't have to. *"Certainly not."* Dignity must be maintained. If you were wealthy enough to fill up on expensive meat and fresh veggies, eating too many stodgy, starchy foods—essentially eating like a Regency peasant—was regarded as a marked stoop from your lofty seat of luxury. And nothing, as Emma reminds us, is worse than being mistaken for "a completely gross, vulgar farmer." Obviously mortifying.

The prejudice was sweeping and widespread. In his classic 1775 dictionary, Dr. Johnson couldn't even define *oats* without a touch of requisite carb snobbery. Oats are "a grain," he says, clearly suppressing a laugh, "which in England is generally given to horses, but in [poorer] Scotland supports the people."[1] No wonder Austen is so careful to define carbs properly too. In *Emma*, rich Mr. Woodhouse might "relish" an evening bowl of "gruel" (made with boiled oats), but Austen repeatedly reminds us that this is extra-special, rich-people gruel, "smooth" and "thin," served in small quantities—a "small basin of thin gruel . . . was all that he could . . . recommend." In other words, Mr. Woodhouse's gruel is a dainty, oat-flavored, almost drinkable nightcap; by no means a solid form of sustenance.

Cookbooks of the era subliminally reinforced the idea. In the best-selling *The Art of Cookery Made Plain and Easy* (1747) with its list of nearly four hundred recommended menu items to choose from, only 10 percent of the dishes would be considered "carb heavy." These were things like rice pudding, apple dumplings, meat pies, and that crazy new noodle import from Italy—macaroni. There was always bread too, at breakfast, but as we've already seen, the English gentry were careful to enjoy their slices as refined and thin as possible. Few dared to eat past this social starch limit. Those who did discovered that carbing-out proved problematic in more ways than one.

"Starched Notions"

As much as us moderns might like to attribute the revolutionary "discovery" that carbs tend to make people fat to the late twentieth century, it was rather old news to history. People had long made the causal link. It wasn't just unfashionable to eat like a ploughing peasant, it was physically infeasible. Only those doing the sweaty, "dirty and nasty" manual jobs seemed to be able to eat lots of carbs without consequences. For everyone else—the elegant rich folk sitting more than sweating—carbs made them pack on the pounds.

The first to put it in writing was the French epicure Brillat-Savarin in 1825. Penning one of history's first diet books—*The Physiology of Taste*—Brillat-Savarin singled out carbs as "the principal cause of obesity" for the rich and well-to-do. His fattest friends, he noticed, were the ones filling up on potatoes, rice, and bread at dinner. Convinced that eating too many "farinaceous foods," "grains and starches," lay at the root of his own weight problem (and his "fairly prominent stomach"), he instructed himself and his readers to dramatically decrease "everything that is starchy or floury" in their diet. "All animals," he said, "who live on farinaceous foods grow fat whether they will or no; man follows the common rule."[2]

Austen would have grown up observing this "common rule" in action. Her dad was a part-time farmer (a respectable farmer, mind you, not a "completely gross, vulgar" one), and it was a well-established trick of the agricultural trade. When farmers throughout England wanted to quickly fatten up their livestock for market, they didn't feed them fat but grains. Lots of grains—the easiest way to plump up your peaky-looking cow, pig, or chicken.[3] And like Brillat-Savarin, Austen knew this applied to people too. The evidence is in *Emma*.

Throughout the novel, Jane Fairfax eats very little, grows thin, and eventually stops eating entirely during a stress-snap over her secret engagement to Frank

Churchill. Poor Jane, "appetite quite gone." People are concerned she's liable to waste away. So problem-solver Emma Woodhouse gears into action, immediately turning to the one food guaranteed to get Jane back to her former, "most becoming" size and weight: carbs. Arrowroot, in this case. Essentially pure starch (like cornstarch, to be made into a thick, filling pudding), a present of "arrowroot" is quickly dispatched to Jane with Emma's full confidence that it will do the trick, returning Jane to her beautiful, buxom self. Within half an hour, however, "the arrowroot was returned" uneaten with a note from Jane that sizzles with indignant offense. Apparently, the woman isn't terribly flattered at being treated like an underfed Regency cow.

Soon, thousands of miles away, another nineteenth-century writer would make the same carb/weight connection. In Leo Tolstoy's Russian novel *Anna Karenina*, Count Vronsky is training for the horse races and must, therefore, stay in fine fettle in order to compete. "He had to avoid gaining weight," says Tolstoy, so naturally "he avoided starchy foods."[4]

To Austen, Tolstoy, and Brillat-Savarin, being carb cautious was part instinct, part snobbery, and part dietary wisdom. Though if you're failing to grasp the connection yourself, here's a quick brush-up on the science behind the historic logic.

A carb-heavy diet was so helpful in giving Regency peasants the power to plough a field because carbs quickly transform into sugar in the body. Sugar is an excellent source of instant energy, fueling muscles to make all necessary furrows in said field. In this way, carbs have provided a vital energy boost to humanity for thousands of years. Yet the very energy-boosting power of carbs causes a problem when people, like the vast population of Austenworld, put down their ploughs and turn them into dainty parasols. Eating a carb-heavy peasant diet when you're not, well, sweatin' like a peasant (somebody please make an exercise video under that title forthwith) means you're taking in far more sugar energy than you can realistically burn off. The result: excess sugar energy in the body always gets transformed into fat.

Dr. Grant offers living proof in *Mansfield Park*. Not only is he lazy and inactive, he also has quite a big carb tooth. Afternoons at the parsonage will usually find him "doing the honors" to a large tray of carb-rich sandwiches. The combination isn't a good one. Dr. Grant is the chubbiest character in Jane's novels.

But before you jump to any carb-free extremes, let's hear Austen out.

Jane was *not* a preincarnate, wittier, and prettier version of Dr. Atkins. She never did anything as dreary and soul-depressing as counting carbs or taking the tops off of sandwiches (in case she was offered one by Dr. Grant). But she did leave us with what's probably the best and most natural strategy for living with carbs in the long run: eat carbs ("grains and starches") according to your activity level.

You'll find Austen frequently repeating this advice. When her characters' energy levels rise, carbs are meted out more freely in her novels. After the cardio workout of a Regency ball, Mrs. Weston proposes "sandwiches" for a respectable energy boost. And after the "healthy . . . benefit of a country run," the Knightly boys hasten home where an Austen-approved bowl of "rice pudding" is waiting for them.

These have always been the best times to carb indulge: during days when your activity level ensures more sugar burning than fat storing, when you are, essentially, behaving more like a physically active peasant. However, on days when you're doing a "Dr. Grant" (sitting, working on your Sunday sermon, what have you), it's best to stay away from "the sandwich tray" and keep carbs to a minimum, filling up instead on the wealthier Regency alternatives—meat and veggies.

Simply put, get your Regency snob on. Put a little dignity back into your "starched notions." Refuse, as Emma says, to be "confined to the society of the illiterate and vulgar all your life!" And for heaven's sake, stop looking so smug about that quinoa.

Rice Pudding

Serves 4

"Their . . . healthy, glowing faces showed all the benefit of a country run, and seemed to ensure a quick dispatch of the roast mutton and rice pudding they were hastening home for."
—*Emma*

Imported from the East, rice was one of the more expensive starches during the Regency era, making it fashionable enough to get an honorable mention in *Emma*.

INGREDIENTS

1 cup water	½ cup long-grain rice
1 cinnamon stick	1 cup half and half
Pinch of salt	¼ cup heavy cream
4 tablespoons sugar, divided	⅛ teaspoon vanilla extract

1. Put the water, cinnamon stick, salt, and 3 tablespoons of the sugar in a medium saucepan. Bring to a boil over high heat. Stir in the rice, reduce heat to low, cover the saucepan, and cook until the rice is tender and the water is absorbed, about 20 minutes.

2. Pour in the half and half and continue to simmer, stirring frequently, until the liquid is thickened and creamy, about 15 minutes. Remove the cinnamon stick and discard.

3. Stir in the heavy cream, vanilla extract, and remaining 1 tablespoon of sugar. Cook and stir for a couple of minutes until thickened and creamy again. Serve warm or cover and refrigerate until chilled.

"I advise you to go out: the air will do you good."

—*Mansfield Park*

6

"A TASTE FOR NATURE"

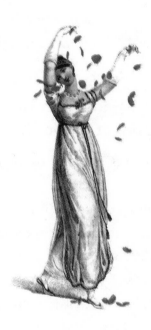

The surprise of finding a "nature" chapter in a diet book may be considerable, so you're free to let out a confused grumble if it helps: *"Surprises are foolish things. The pleasure is not enhanced, and the inconvenience is often considerable."*

Trust me, I certainly wasn't expecting it myself. Writing a Jane Austen diet book, I imagined, would confine me to the usual spheres of food and fitness—the solid things you can put a fork or foot to. Jane would play along like a good girl, approaching "health" as nothing more than the right way to eat and exercise. Things, err, didn't go as planned . . .

Jane refused the scheme outright, kept insisting nature was important, we had a terrible fight, I said some nasty things about "Regency tree-hugging" and "not in my book!" then stumped off to do some research. At which point I ate a huge slice of humble pie. As usual, Austen was right.

"She Had Often Great Enjoyment Out of Doors"

Admittedly, her nudges are hard to miss. Austen practically tattoos I ♥ NATURE over all her heroines' chests. The sensual delights of nature, of fresh air, woods, gardens, sunshine, and shade: they pop up more reliably than Austen's leading men. "What are young men to rocks and mountains?" asks Lizzie, joking-not-joking to her sister that she fell in love with Darcy only *after* "seeing his beautiful grounds at Pemberley." Happiness is only complete in Austenworld if it comes with an attached garden to stroll through. An entire "park" with its own river and "ten miles" of winding wooded walks, even better.

"Elizabeth longed to explore its windings"—a longing for nature shared by every healthy body from *Pride and Prejudice* to *Persuasion*. Whether that's a walk around the shrubbery, a whiff of sea air, a sparkle of sunlight, or a twinkle of stars on a clear night, Austen characters gulp it all down like an essential vitamin, as much a part of a wholesome diet as three meals a day. It's a world where simply breathing in "fresh air" is a pharmaceutical drug, where the more you languish indoors, the more everyone will strongly "advise you to go out," where lolloping through muddy fields and looking "almost wild" is a good thing.

In a word, Austenworld is teeming with *biophilia*—the belief that our bodies (being a part of nature) need frequent, physical contacts with nature in order to thrive.[1] And I can say that straight faced, without wearing dreadlocks, smoking a joint, or seeing Jupiter align with Mars. The best minds of ancient Greece believed in the health benefits of nature, Austen believed it, I've personally experienced it, and science now confirms it. Like Fanny in *Mansfield Park*, all of us have an innate "taste for nature" imprinted on our DNA—a missing puzzle piece to physical and mental well-being found, free of charge, just outside our front doors. Our current techno-driven detachment from nature might give us more reasons to look up from our screens and remember Austen's insights, but the fundamentals remain the same. In Mansfield Park or modern suburbia, our relationship to the environment—to natural light, air, earth, and darkness—has always been vital to our relationship to better health.

"A Bright Morning"

We'll begin with mornings in Austenworld, something I used to chalk up as pure Regency fluff. If you haven't already noticed, the place is overrun with morning people gone mad. The sort of people who pop out of bed and instantly start praising the "lovely," "cheerful," "charming morning"—who rush into other people's bedrooms, throw open the shutters, and scream "Make haste!" The sort of lovable sap reinforced by the opening film sequence of *Pride and Prejudice* (2005)—cue the birdsong, the piano music trilling in the background, the sun rising in the distance, and—oh, look! There's Lizzie out in a nearby field, reading, walking, smirking, effortlessly multitasking at the break of dawn. Of course she is, the dear.

One either sighs or seethes at such blatant suspensions from modern reality—the squinty-eyed-slump-to-the-coffee-maker sort of reality (what Jane would call "the staggers"). And I, for one, staggered with the worst before realizing all of Austenworld is smirking with Lizzie for good reason. They're all in on one of the biggest secrets to waking up with "natural cheerfulness." And Jane hides it in plain sight.

In every novel, Austen characters are famous for rolling out of bed and, almost immediately, rushing outside. Lizzie makes a three-mile dash across country fields before Bingley has even sat down to breakfast. Then there's Anne and Henrietta, strolling "down to the sea before breakfast" in *Persuasion*, or Jane Fairfax on her usual walk to the post office "before breakfast" in *Emma*, or Colonel Brandon's frequent rambles to Barton Cottage, "early enough . . . before breakfast" in *Sense and Sensibility*. How do they find the energy? we ask. How do *they* have energy without it? they'd respond. "A walk before breakfast does me good," says Jane Fairfax. "I am advised to be out of doors as much as I can."

The calculation comes easy to Austen characters (morning + outdoors = feel good) because they lived in a world that respected a truth most of us have forgotten. Little wonder: waking up in dark bedrooms, swigging coffee in dim kitchens, and driving to work in tinted cars would sap the wits out of any Austenite. These are people literally made brighter by "a bright morning."

We all are, in fact. If you're human (not vampire), you're automatically *diurnal*, a creature of daylight—to rise with the rhythm of the sun is powerfully built into your biology. Morning light isn't just nice, we *need* it to stay healthy. It's a symbiotic relationship. As morning light fills the sky, light receptors in our eyes trigger important "new day" signals in our bodies, keeping our own natural rhythms—heart, brain, metabolism, appetite, weight, mood, energy—in proper working order.[2] The sickening effects of jet lag, for instance, is caused when these rhythms are disrupted for only a day. Yet even mild disruptions of morning light will leave us feeling like we're hobbling along on the wrong side of a Regency zombie novel.

However, getting outside and exposing our eyes to natural morning light immediately tells our brains to stop pumping out melatonin—the hormone responsible for making us feel groggy and dead tired. Vital for a good night's sleep, melatonin can be a real downer if allowed to continue pumping into the morning, keeping us in that sluggish, unshakeable sleep mode even if our eyes are wide open. Surrounding ourselves with morning sunshine, however—even on a cloudy day—will stop melatonin production in its tracks. The same morning-light signal which simultaneously releases another important hormone—cortisol. Melatonin's energetic twin, cortisol is like a biological shot of espresso, the daytime hormone making you feel active and fully alert.[3]

Flipping these hormonal switches is as easy as flooding your eyes with natural light. It begins by throwing open your bedroom shutters as soon as you wake up. Luckier characters in Austenworld have housemaids for that purpose ("the housemaid's folding back her window-shutters at eight o'clock the next day was the sound which first roused Catherine"). So either hire a maid, enlist a willing child, or do it yourself. Then head outside as soon as possible. Even the light on overcast days is ten times brighter than artificial indoor lighting,[4] waking you up quicker and more naturally than any energy drink you could ever swig. A leisurely stroll is all Austen advises. Exercise isn't the main priority here. Anne and Henrietta are relaxedly "loitering about" on their morning walk in *Persuasion*. The real goal is to give your body the opportunity to respond to "the return of day"—energy and spunk will automatically follow. "I cannot give up my early walk," confesses Jane Fairfax. And neither should any of us. It's always been the fastest, healthiest way to wake up fully alive. Besides, hearing that lovely piano music trilling in the background is always a nice bonus. It can't be just me!

Regency Alarm Clocks

Beep! Beep! Beep!—it is not a noise Austen was "at all acquainted with." So throw out that modern alarm clock, "all clamorous, and impertinent," and switch to the calmer sounds Jane would have awoken to. Birdsong, in particular, filled the English countryside at daybreak, flowing into every bedroom in Austenworld. Beginning at dawn and rising in a gentle crescendo, the sprightly songs of robins, blackbirds, and sparrows were nature's soft reminders of "the return of day" and the "cheerfulness of morning." Even today, waking up to bird sounds (either real or recorded) has been shown to boost mood and reduce fatigue.[5] As the universal music of morning, we seem hardwired to respond pleasantly to these chirping cues to wake up. The jolting beeps of a typical alarm clock, on the other hand, can be a literal jolt to your system: elevating your blood pressure and stress levels before getting out of bed.[6] Not a difficult choice to make. *"Shall any of us object to being comfortable?"*

"Sparkling Vivacity"

Let's linger a little longer over Austen's relationship with sunshine, the beams of which brighten her entire romantic

universe. Generations of readers have felt the almost palpable warmth emanating from *Pride and Prejudice*, one
of those rare books that literally feels, from start to finish,
like a sunshiny day. Austen was the first to agree. If *Pride
and Prejudice* had one fault, she teased her sister in 1813,
it was "rather too light, and bright, and sparkling" for its
own good. Lord David Cecil later swung the point home:
People who do not like Jane Austen are the sort of people
"who do not like sunshine."[7]

You can set your meteorological watches by it. When
the sun is out, so is everybody else in Austenworld. As
Catherine observes in *Northanger Abbey*, a sunny day
unfailingly "empties every house of its inhabitants, and all
the world appears on such an occasion to walk about and
tell their acquaintance what a charming day it is." The
mere "promise of sunshine" in Jane's novels is enough to
plan picnics, go on long drives in the country, or enjoy
a few more turns around the garden, a mood perfectly
reflected in Marianne's "felicity" in the 1995 film version
of *Sense and Sensibility*. Drenched with rain and dragging
Margaret up a muddy hilltop, she spots the merest glint of
sunshine in the distance: "Look! There is some blue sky!
Let us chase it!"[8]

Being honest, few of us chase sunbeams with the same
happy exuberance nowadays. Sunshine, peered through
a modern lens, isn't exactly the many-splendored thing
it was for Jane. Most of us no longer know what a healthy
relationship with the sun looks like—or if it's even healthy

at all—a cultural question mark that might have already convinced you that really healthy people are just the sort Lord Cecil dreaded: the kind of people "who do not like sunshine" period.

You can blame it on the 1960s (I know I do for everything), an era when moderation knew no bounds, especially when it came to the sun. All those teenie-weenie polka-dot bikinis, all that tanning oil, all those inordinate hours sunbathing semi-naked did what most things do when frequently abused: it made some people sick (and made other people just look plain awful). Fears of sun cancer and the sun's effect on aging quickly followed, pushing our cultural pendulum far enough for an inevitably dizzy swing back. Now "smart" people are solar-phobic: skittishly looking for nooks of shade wherever they go, or squirting on sunscreen just for a drive to the mall, or generally seeing the sun as a nuclear death ray in the sky. Reader, I was one of "these poor creatures," and am now in steady recovery thanks to Jane. The infomercial of my life proves Lord Cecil was right: you can't read Austen and hate the sun at the same time. Or, more importantly, not appreciate its amazing benefits.

"Gaiety in Sunshine"

A helpful reminder is that only silly, prissy, petty people—permanent parasols-up-their-butts sort of characters (pardon my Regency French)—have a problem with the sun in Jane's novels. Caroline Bingley in *Pride and Prejudice* can't even look at Lizzie's ever-so-slight summer tan without scoffing up ridiculous exaggerations: "How very ill Eliza Bennet looks . . . I never in my life saw anyone so much altered . . . She is grown so brown and coarse!" Her fellow solar-phobe in arms is Sir Walter in *Persuasion*—a pallid prig who considers anyone that actually likes the sun personally "offensive": "they are all knocked about, and exposed . . . till they are not fit to be seen. It is a pity they are not knocked on the head at once." Yet the real ironic pity is that these people could loosen up by getting a bit more of the thing they loathe. Because as everyone else in Austenworld knows, sunlight is truly the stuff of happiness. Fanny describes it as the hidden "gaiety in sunshine" in *Mansfield Park*, a physical sense that sunlight literally lifts the spirits—one of the most verified sensations in the books:

- As the sun "appeared" on the picnic party in *Sense and Sensibility*, "they were all in high spirits and good humour."
- "A gleam of sunshine" in *Northanger Abbey* makes Catherine correspondingly "happy."
- "The sun appeared" and Emma's "spirits freshened."

You probably have sensed it yourself. A day at the beach usually leaves people running high on euphorically good feelings (and accounting for why most of us prefer holidays in sunny locales over, say, the Arctic Tundra—a preference that's quite literally all in our heads). Sunlight triggers our brains to produce more of the feel-good chemical serotonin—the hormone that helps balance and better our moods, the same hormone drug companies now pop into antidepressants. "More sunlight meant better moods," confirmed a pivotal study in 2002, "less sunlight led to symptoms of depression."[9]

Pfft. Austen had already figured *that* out in 1814. When her brother Edward was stressed out and shut up indoors from wintry weather, Austen nails the perfect remedy—"Edward's spirits will be wanting sunshine." How much our own bodies want sunshine is still being researched, its refracted benefits reaching far beyond mood. Since 1984, for instance, doctors have noticed that patients recovering from surgery in hospital rooms with sunny window views (rather than just looking at brick walls) had shorter hospital stays and needed less pain medication.[10] Brightening our days with a bit of sunlight also gives us better sleep, better bones, and better eyesight, causing health experts worldwide to push back on the pendulum. Today, "responsible sun exposure" is the new "run for your lives to the shade!" Just the moderate sun prescription Austen advised all along.

You won't find any lobster-red sun worshippers among her heroines. The sun's healing warmth, like everything else in Austenworld, needs its counter dose of "cooling moderation." Too much and you risk looking like the sun-beaten Admiral Baldwin in *Persuasion*: "his face the colour of mahogany, rough and rugged to the last degree, all lines and wrinkles." Too little sun and you'll join the sallow ranks of Miss de Bourgh in *Pride and Prejudice*: "pale and sickly" and about as attractive to Darcy as a porcelain chamber pot. Yet striking the perfect balance is what Austen's heroines do best—"sparkling in sunshine and freshness" without overdoing it (and all without sunscreen). Here's how:

Timing. Not all sunlight is "cheerful" in Austenworld. In fact, the intense glare of midday sun is positively "insufferable." In *Emma*, the strawberry pickers soon stop picking once "the glaring sun" comes out, all saying they "could bear it no longer—must go sit in the shade," a feeling shared by the walking party at Sotherton in *Mansfield Park*. Finding the midday sun "insufferably hot," they head for the "darkness and shade" of a nearby wood, "leaving the unmitigated glare of day behind." It's still one of the best solar secrets to copy today. The sun's UV radiation is strongest at midday, a time when the sun isn't just hotter and higher in sky, its skin damaging potential is higher too. Austen characters, instead, prefer to be outside in more "amiable light." Mornings and late afternoons are the usual times for sauntering outdoors in Jane's novels—appropriately enough, times when the sun's UV rays are always gentlest and safest.

Protection. Of course, there are times in Austenworld (oh, say, an impromptu visit from Lady Catherine) when characters are forced to face the sun at inconvenient times. And at such moments, even sun-loving Lizzie reaches "for her parasol." Parasols, bonnets, hats—these are the sunscreens of Regency life. And while I don't necessarily recommend all of the above today—especially walking outside with a parasol/umbrella when it's *not* raining (rude people in cars tend to stare and shout garbled threats—I know from personal experience)—there are benefits to following the general spirit. Hats and clothing are usually better at blocking the sun than slathering on sunscreen. They act as physical shields to the sun's rays, whereas sunscreen is applied to exposed skin (and often not correctly). That is, *rubbing* a thin layer of sunscreen into the skin (as opposed to keeping a thick, buttery layer on top) can do more harm than good. When the chemicals in most modern sunscreens are absorbed into the skin, they inadvertently allow the sun's rays to absorb deeper as well, increasing the risk of skin damage and premature aging.[11] Better to do a Regency rethink: donning your own modern version of "a very smart bonnet" when you'd rather stay out of the sun.

"The Shades of Pemberley"

Jane Austen was cool enough *without* sunglasses, *"perfectly so, I thank you."* And it might be time to ditch the shades ourselves. Designed to inhibit light, sunglasses do it a bit too well, blocking our eyes from experiencing the natural light needed to trigger important, healthy hormone secretions in our bodies. "We must allow for the effect of shade," says

Austen, and shading our eyes at inappropriate times could even be damaging. Sunglasses circumvent a very protective optical talent. Without sunglasses, our eyes naturally know how to shield themselves from the sun's UV rays. Bright light automatically causes our pupils to shrink, drastically limiting their sun exposure. Dim light does the opposite: opening our pupils wide to let in as much light as possible. Sunglasses confuse this natural reflex, tricking our eyes into thinking the sun has already set on a shady world. Our pupils are subsequently left wide open, potentially letting in harmful UV rays, just when they should be shrinking.[12] But nobody need squint while Jane's around. Her historically safer alternative: "Put on your hat this moment."

"We Are So Remarkably Airy!"

Ah, the heady delights of "fresh air"—Austen's most shamelessly convenient plot device.

It's easier to count the number of heroines who *don't* bump into men after popping outside for the innocent "enjoyment of air." *None.* Marianne's own tale is condensed into something like: need fresh air—there's a hilltop—let's climb it—sprain an ankle—meet Willoughby—go bonkers—nearly die—end of story. And yet, "fresh air" in Jane's novels is pretty neat stuff in its own right. You might even call it Austenworld's recreational drug of choice.

Purely "breathing fresh air is enough" to put a rosy glow, a happy smile, and a spring in the step of her characters— outdoor "air" and physical "ecstasies" being one and the same. Literal airheads, the lot of them. "We are so very airy!" brags Isabella Knightley in *Emma*. "Air" even winds up on their pharmaceutical prescriptions. Jane Fairfax only enters the neighborhood of Highbury under the strict orders from an offstage doctor, prescribing she dose up on more country "air, for the recovery of her health." What *are* these people puffing? Incidentally, the same fresh air we should all be puffing more on.

Think back to the last time you turned off the AC and opened all the windows in your house, or the last time you drove on a country road with the windows rolled down, letting the breeze fly freely in your face. Chances are you felt a weird and wonderful sense of physical well-being, stretching your arm out the window in response, riding your fingers up and down on the flittering wind (the human equivalent of a dog dangling its tongue out the car window). It's a universal instinct. Back in the 1940s, the British government knew there was something inherently healthy in fresh air, advising housewives during WWII to step outside for frequent "air baths" whenever they could. Mothers in modern Scandinavia are likewise famous for their staunch belief in the curative benefits of fresh air, actually *preferring* their children nap outdoors, even in the middle of winter. Japan's "forest bathing" movement is now one of the country's most powerful pillars of preventative healthcare, involving nothing more than a slow, airy walk through the woods. And so we circle back to Jane, who predicted it three centuries ago: that we are all made "materially better for change of air"—a mysterious relationship with an invisible element no heroine's (or human's) health is complete without.

Long before we sealed off our homes from the outside world, Austen knew that indoor and outdoor air were two different things. Inside air could go stale, or "foul," as Austen sensed it. Regency homes had their own air-quality issues.[13] Soot and smoke from fireplaces meant the air not only smelled differently inside, it made people *feel* differently too. Austen characters often complain of a mysterious "dullness" whenever they're cooped up indoors for too long. In *Pride and Prejudice*, Jane Bennet does "not look well" after a prolonged period inside. Staying indoors is likewise the worst punishment Mr. Bennet can inflict on poor Kitty: "You are never to stir out of doors till you can prove that you have spent ten minutes of every day in a rational manner." "How horrid all this is!" cries Charlotte Palmer in *Sense and Sensibility*, going stir-crazy when only one day of rain keeps her shut up indoors. "Such weather makes everything and everybody disgusting."

"She Ought Never to Be Long Banished from the Free Air"

Today, we'd recognize these odd symptoms as "sick building syndrome"—as in, why most people feel inexplicably lousy (in health, mood, or general well-being) the more time they spend indoors. And it's far more consequential now than it ever was for Austen. Modern buildings contain more than just Regency fires to "foul" up the air. Synthetic chemicals in our paints, flooring, furniture, bedding, plastics, cleaning supplies, and air "fresheners" make for more *indoor* pollution than even Fanny in *Mansfield Park* could imagine. She physically slumps by just being in a stuffy house in Portsmouth: "she was in the midst of closeness . . . confinement, bad air, bad smells." And most of us are slumping today without realizing it. In 2004, Danish researchers found that being near the volatile fumes emitted by modern computers can negatively affect how people think and concentrate.[14] All more reason to embrace Austen's smart solution: popping outside for a "pleasant airing" whenever you can. "I advise you to go out: the air will do you good."

Stepping outside is enough to "comfort" Anne, "tranquilize" Fanny, "freshen" Emma, and "inspire" Marianne—observations incredibly attuned to scientific reality. Fresh air recharges our mental batteries because it's literally energized differently than indoor air. Unlike the tightly sealed, stagnant air inside our homes, the constantly circulating air outside ("the free air," as Austen calls it) means it's a naturally abundant source of supercharged negative ions.[15] Negative ions are the antioxidants of the air—the more we breathe, the better we feel. Science is still discovering how they do it, but negative ions seem to instantly improve our ability to absorb and transport oxygen throughout our brain and body, resulting in an elevated sense of physical and mental well-being. This is the unique "property" of fresh air that Charlotte from *Sanditon* fundamentally believes in: "It has always some property that is wholesome and invigorating to me."

It's unsurprising, then, that places with the highest negative-ion counts, where air and water churn about most freely (at the seaside, for instance), are the places people feel at their best. Just listen to the happy holidayers at the beachside town of Lyme in *Persuasion*: "Oh! yes, I am quite convinced that . . . the sea-air always does good. There can be no doubt of its having been of the greatest service to Dr. Shirley, after his illness . . . He declares himself, that coming to Lyme for a month, did him more good than all the medicine he took; and, that being by the sea, always makes him feel young again."

Most of us can get the same feeling closer to home. After rainstorms, for instance, the air tingles with higher negative-ion counts.[16] Emma seems to be innately aware of it, eagerly soaking up the energized air after a heavy summer storm: "In the afternoon it cleared" and "Emma resolved to be out of doors as soon as possible. Never had the exquisite sight, smell, sensation of nature, tranquil, warm, and brilliant after a storm, been more attractive to her." And there, her "spirits freshened."

But then again, even Emma can't be running about all day chasing ionized raindrops. The woman has better things to do (paint Harriet's picture, *frame* Harriet's picture, ruin love lives, the list goes on and on). We feel ya, Emma—life is "rather busy" for all of us, so it's always handy to keep a few other fresh-air strategies up your muslin sleeve:

1. "I Am Very Fond of Standing at an Open Window"

Simply opening a nearby window can do wonders in improving the indoor air quality. It's truly the healthiest air "freshener" at our disposal, according to researchers at the University of Leeds, who found that opening windows in hospital rooms dramatically reduces the risk of infection.[17] Germs, fungal spores, carbon dioxide, and noxious fumes from electronic gadgets abound in buildings that are tightly shut-in from the "free air" outside, which would compel Mr. Woodhouse to point out, "I told you so!" Rooms that are "never properly aired" are "dangerous," he says in *Emma*—stale air being his prime concern for holding a ball at the long-stagnant rooms of the Crown Inn. Yet all is soon put to rights and the health of Highbury restored by—what else?—the promise that its windows would soon be open and the ballroom "thoroughly aired."

2. "I Hope You Have Had a Pleasant Airing"

Austenites love a good "airing," Jane's term for joy-riding in an open carriage, the Regency equivalent of driving in the car with the windows down. And seeing that we now spend more time in our modern carriages than ever before, it isn't off the health mark to say along with Mrs. Bennet, "an airing would do me a great deal of good." Because unless you're sitting in the gassy smog of bumper-to-bumper traffic, the air outside your vehicle is undeniably fresher than the air inside. The ACs in our cars are notorious for circulating unwanted microbes and bacteria in confined spaces. Eight types of mold were found living in the air-conditioning systems of the cars tested by researchers at Louisiana State Medical Center.[18] And as for that lovely "new car smell," it's nothing less than toxic, a two-hundred-plus-chemical attack that can cause everything from headaches to hormonal imbalances.[19] So roll down those windows because here comes Miss Bates: "Miss Bates came to the carriage door, all gratitude, and agreeing with her most earnestly in thinking an airing might be of the greatest service."

3. "To the Copse"

Regency estates weren't complete without "copses"—woodland retreats where heroines idly roam and find near magical "refreshment" amongst the trees. A wooded grove brings instant "comfort" to Anne's cluttered mind in *Persuasion*, and Lizzie finds inexpressible "enjoyment" under the tree-lined path boarding the Rosings estate. Marianne waxes poetic when remembering her autumnal walks in Norland's woods: "How have I delighted, as I walked . . .

What feelings have they, the season, the air altogether inspired!" Interestingly, the same sensations are now associated with one of the biggest health trends in modern Japan. *Shinrin-yoku* ("forest bathing") is the belief that a leisurely stroll through the woods is deeply rejuvenating for the body and mind. Forest air is particularly rich in phytoncides—fragrant, antimicrobial compounds swirling around trees that, when inhaled, can reduce stress and boost our immune system. Spending time among trees specifically elevates our "NK" cells (white blood cells that fight tumors and infections), according to a seminal Japanese study.[20] And most of us have a Regency-style "copse" in easy distance—whether it's a wooded park or the backwoods just beyond our backyards. There, like Fanny, we can substitute the "bad air, bad smells" of indoor life "for liberty, freshness, fragrance, and verdure."

"Oh! . . . I Never Mind Dirt"

Don't be afraid of good clean dirt. Lizzie certainly isn't. She splashes about in mud on her walk to Netherfield Park, bearing her soiled hems with pride. The evil Bingley sisters are evidently disgusted—"She really looked almost wild . . . I hope you saw her petticoat, six inches deep in mud." Today, they'd be squirting bottles of hand sanitizer down Lizzie's throat if they could—though Lizzie could easily outwit them. In fact, living with a more relaxed attitude toward dirt can give us all clearer heads. Getting a bit dirty gets us in contact with the "friendly" bacteria in soil, particularly *Mycobacterium vaccae*. Usually inhaled whenever people potter about in dirt, *M. vaccae* reduces anxiety by boosting the positive brain chemical serotonin in ways very similar to antidepressant pills.[21] Garden soil and garden air has always been the best source of this natural high. Charlotte Palmer is clearly a happy soil sniffer in *Sense and Sensibility*. Merely strolling through the gardens and greenhouses at Cleveland "raised the laughter of Charlotte" to giddy heights.

"I Am Quite in the Dark"

As night falls on Austenworld, Jane's nature prescription comes full circle. Meaning, the residual bonus of soaking up more natural light and fresh air during the day is the amazing sleep it can give us at night—the sort of deep "slumber" Marianne sinks body and heart into, rising "the next morning with recovered spirits and happy looks." Or the "sound sleep" Catherine "immediately fell into," lasting "nine hours, and from which she awoke perfectly revived, in excellent spirits, with fresh hopes and fresh schemes." Though if you really want to sleep like Austenworld's romantically reclined—enjoying the full body "cure" of "a good night's rest"—you'll need to reacquaint yourself with the Regency rhythms and natural essence of night itself: darkness.

Darkness isn't exactly the top buzzword associated with Jane Austen nowadays. Thanks to Hollywood magic, most of us now picture Regency nightlife as an endless round of bright ballrooms for busting a move under a million-watt chandelier. But the truth requires we turn down the dimmer a bit. As Austen verifies, hers was "a much darker night."

No electricity, street lamps in the country, or glares from television sets meant that when it got *dark* in Regency England, it was truly literal. And almost palpable. In *Northanger Abbey*, night brings "darkness impenetrable" to the world. The same "immovable" darkness prevents the ladies from venturing outside in *Persuasion*: "The nights were too dark for the ladies to meet again till the morrow." Firelight and candles were the only countering luminescence inside, making the helpful glow of moonlight so "delightfully" important to Jane and her contemporaries. The best Regency balls were only held on full-moon nights, ensuring the partygoers could travel safely to and fro under its silvery light.[22] Sir John, for instance, can't rustle up any last-minute company in *Sense and Sensibility* for just this reason: because "it was moonlight and everybody was [already] full of engagements." For most of Jane's life, nights never got much brighter than what nature allowed under a full moon. *"There are undoubtedly many who could not say the same . . ."*

If you want a visual of how utterly un-Regency our nights have become, take that globe-looking thing spinning in Gwyneth Paltrow's hand in *Emma* (1996), pop a flashlight in, then jab it with about a billion tiny dots. That's basically what our nocturnal world looks like from outer space. We are "splendidly lit up," as Austen would say, though scientists would more bluntly label it, "light pollution." More than half the world's population lives under a nightly sky brighter than the brightest full moon.[23] And it's not just harder to see the many stars Fanny easily spots on clear nights at Mansfield Park.

The average home at night now beams with the equivalent of hundreds of Regency candles. LED lights, televisions, iPads, and phone screens all fill our eyes with what would only be considered by Austen as an "overpowering, blinding, bewildering" amount of nighttime illumination. Sure, we've gotten used to it. Our eyes have adjusted, and darkness or dimness is only a switch we flick right before we hop into bed. But if we listen to Jane (and science) we're using darkness—or rather, not using it—all wrong.

"The Evening Is Closing In"

First, the darkening night sky *should* compel our bodies to wind down. Natural darkness was an "impenetrable" barrier to how much work Austenites could accomplish at night. This was Jane's "closing in" time: when shutters were drawn, candles were lit, and people settled in for "a quiet evening." Balls, of course, were periodically attended and "moonlight walks" in summer a special treat, but by and large, this was no occasion for serious exercise or work. General Tilney's insistence that he must work late into the night at his desk in *Northanger Abbey* is markedly odd and "not very likely" to Catherine. There simply wasn't enough light to make it productive. Austen speaks of the rosy "dimness" of Regency candles. They emitted enough light for the usual "evening amusements" of Austenworld—reading, playing card games, or music—but not enough to get, too often, much wilder than that. Yawns gradually commence and by 10:00 p.m., the majority of Austenworld is ready for bed.

Today, most of us only experience this Regency nighttime ritual on camping trips. As the sun sets, and with only the amber light from a fire, our bodies instinctually settle down, popping into sleeping bags far earlier and more tired than usual. Normally, however, "closing in" at night means clicking on. Bright lights and even brighter screens mean we can now work and exercise at whatever hour we wish, though ignoring the cues of darkness comes with unintended consequences—sickness, for one. Working too frequently at night is now listed as a "suspected carcinogen" by the American Cancer Society.[24] The biological stress involved in overriding your body's natural desire to wind down at night can wreak havoc on your immune system—not to mention your sleep quality, as Austen well knew. Being too busy or stressed at night is the one thing guaranteed to keep Austen characters up and buzzing. "I have passed a wretched night," says Marianne, stressed out by the scoundrel Willoughby. And when that happens, Austenites rely on that same old-fashioned darkness to wind them back down again.

"Lord, How Tired I Am!"

Personally, I don't think it's a coincidence that Austen's darkest book, the faux-mystery novel *Northanger Abbey*, is also her only book to use the term "sleeping potion." Natural darkness is indeed the most effective, safest sleeping potion most of us are missing out on. Its nocturnal magic revolves around the aforementioned hormone melatonin—an important brain hormone intimately coupled with the rhythms of night itself. Melatonin helps us relax and unwind, naturally drowsing us up for a good night's sleep. Melatonin is what makes sleep, as Austen says, our "likeliest friend," causing us to fall asleep faster and enjoy deeper slumbers when functioning properly. And that requires dimming our nighttime world to more Regency-appropriate levels.

To use an Austen metaphor, bright lights turn off melatonin like Mr. Collins turns off Lizzie. It's a biological reflex. In nature, bright light (from the sun) is only prevalent during the day: when we *don't* need or want melatonin's drowsy side effects. But when the sun sets—when we *do* need melatonin to calm down—artificial bright lights can delay the whole process, tricking our brains into believing daylight is still going strong. Yes, Regency candles were technically artificial lights too, but they weren't nearly bright enough to turn off melatonin. The same can't be said today. To put our modern nighttime brightness in perspective, flat-screen TVs and computer monitors now emit the light equivalent of four hundred to one thousand Regency candles[25]—more than enough light to suppress melatonin. In a 2014 study conducted by Brigham and Women's Hospital in Boston, simple "screen time" on an iPad at night had far-reaching effects: people secreted less melatonin, took longer to fall asleep, had less restful REM sleep, and felt more tired the following day (despite getting eight hours of sleep).[26]

The top culprit in all of this is blue light. *"We see no blue,"* says Austen. And quite right. Blue light was totally absent from Regency nights, but it's one of our prime illuminators today. Our TVs, computers, and smartphones all emit it: a constant blue glare no matter the colors depicted on the screen. Don't believe me? Stroll around your neighborhood at night and you'll see living-room windows aglow in some shade of blue (actually, never mind, you'll probably look like a creep, so just take my word for it). The basic problem is, blue light doesn't scream "nighttime" to your biology. Quite the opposite. As far as your brain is concerned, blue light means morning light (natural morning light being high in blue wavelengths)— your body's top cue to wake up and start another day, not to wind down after a long one. Melatonin, therefore, gets dramatically suppressed and we end up more habitually wired than Mrs. Bennet: "I am sure I shan't get a wink of sleep all night." This, however, is easily put to rights again by "passing the evening" with more Regency sense:

🏋 Use Austen's "closing in" ritual as a reminder to close down those screens (especially phones and computers) when it gets dark outside. Just two hours of "screen time" before bed is enough to suppress melatonin. Reading an actual printed book under normal lamp-light will not.[27]

🏋 Mr. Woodhouse instructs us to keep "reasonable" hours at night, avoiding stressful work after it gets dark. Few things are "so serious" that you can't tackle tomorrow "with fresh hopes and fresh schemes." And while the occasional late night out is perfectly admissible in Austenworld (Regency balls could keep bouncing until 3:00 a.m.), Jane's characters are usually in bed by 10:00 or 11:00 p.m.

🏋 Emulate the softer glow of Regency candles by switch-ing on dimmer, "warmer" electric lights at nights. Can-dles and traditional low-watt light bulbs both emit rays on the reddish end of the light spectrum: reddish light is associated with sunset in nature, and thus has the least negative effect on melatonin.[28] Fluorescent and LED white lights, however, trick your brain into think-ing it's full daylight again.

🏋 Once in bed, recreate the deeper darkness of Regency nights. After her candle snuffs out, "darkness impen-etrable and immovable filled" Catherine's bedroom in Northanger Abbey. So close tight your curtains and get rid of any unwanted beams of electric light (especially the blue glow from some alarm clocks). Even if your eyes are closed, the photoreceptors on your skin can pick up any ambient light in the room, suppressing melatonin and affecting the overall restfulness of your sleep.[29] *"I would not have you sleep in such an error for the world."*

Regency Stargazing

If nothing else, Austen compels us to remember the easiest nature prescription at our disposal: simply looking at it does a body good. Nature puts things in proper perspective, reminding us to take a breath, that despite the "daily terrors" of life, the earth is still turning and everything will be okay. Gazing at a star-lit night does it for Fanny Price: "When I look out on such a night as this, I feel as if there could be neither wickedness nor sorrow in the world; and there certainly would be less of both if the sublimity of Nature were more attended to, and people were carried more out of themselves by contemplating such a scene." Fanny, you're a genius. Researchers have discovered that nature is such a powerful restorative, even looking at "nature scenes" on a screen can fire up the dopamine reward system in our brains, increasing feelings of wellness, positive thoughts, and a greater drive to form emotional connections with others.[30] No wonder love is in the air in Austenworld!

AUSTEN EATS: GARDEN STUFF

"*Oh! thoughtless, thoughtless, Lydia!*" Lydia being me at the moment. I could kick myself for saving garden stuff for the last Austen Eats chapter. The Regency catch-all term for fruits and vegetables, hitching garden stuff to the back of the line only plays into the old stereotype: that fresh produce was the last-and-certainly-least food on Austen's mind. That somehow, if anything green and leafy wound up on a Regency table, amidst the endless beige of meat, it was an accident, an afterthought, even a joke. After all, the era has never lived down its most infamous veggie one-liner. When Beau Brummell (Regency fashion icon, inventor of the modern suit, wisecracking dandy) was once asked if he liked vegetables, he reflected for a moment, then delivered, "I don't know. I have never eaten them . . . No, that is not quite true. I once ate a pea."[1] But this was a joke, an outrageous exaggeration even in 1800. It didn't reflect how the vast majority of English people felt about their veggies. These earthy edibles were enjoyed, loved, and eaten much more than we might think. Fruit and vegetables not on the Regency radar? "*Believe no such thing . . . Spread no such malicious slander.*" Jane Austen loved her "garden stuff."

"English Verdure . . . English Comfort"

Fresh produce was an integral part of how the "best sort of people" ate in Regency England, as only the best sort of people had money and land to grow as much garden stuff as they liked. In *Sense and Sensibility*, when the Dashwoods leave their palatial home of Norland Park for a raggedy cottage in Devonshire, they also leave behind Norland's vegetable gardens and orchards (and thus their private supply of fresh fruit and vegetables). Sir John quickly recognizes their "deficient" state and sends along "a large basket full of garden stuff" as a cottage consolation present. His soothing symbolic message: Life goes on, ladies. Look on the bright side. You still have vegetables to eat!

You might have noticed the pattern. No sooner do characters visit their rich friends in Austenworld than they're immediately whisked outside to admire the "kitchen garden"—a walled-in lawn of vegetable plots and fruit trees. One's proximity to fresh produce, you see, is quite the legitimate boast in Jane's novels. Mrs. Palmer in *Sense and Sensibility* doesn't begin to do justice to the grandeur of her house until she takes Elinor and Marianne on an ostentatious tour "round the kitchen garden, examining the [fruit] bloom upon its walls" and "dawdling through the green-house." General Tilney dawdles a bit longer. Eager to show off his solid wealth to Catherine, the "unrivaled" kitchen garden at Northanger Abbey does the trick. "The number of acres contained within this garden was such as Catherine could not listen to without dismay . . . The walls seemed countless in number, endless in length; a village of hot-houses seemed to arise among them, and a whole parish to be at work within the enclosure." Encouraged by Catherine's "looks of surprise," the General casually lets it slip that *should* she marry his son Henry, the marriage package will come with an "excellent kitchen garden" of her own. In Jane's novels, conjugal bliss doesn't get much better than constant access to fresh produce. Even the Darcy-dreamboat package gets substantially more blissful once Lizzie beholds "the beautiful pyramids of grapes, nectarines, and peaches" grown fresh in Pemberley's greenhouses. The calculation would have been easy for Austen's original readers to make. Hmm, Mr. Darcy: a man of fruit *and* fortune. Yep, Lizzie is going up in the world.

The arc of Jane's own story follows an identical pattern. During good times, fresh produce grew steps from her back door. During bad times, it was much harder to come by. Her childhood and adolescence (undoubtedly the most financially secure periods of her life) came with the luxury of living in a comfy rectory in Hampshire with two walled gardens bursting with fruit and vegetables. But a substantial drop in income and a subsequent move to the city center of Bath made fresh produce scarce for a time. In Bath, Jane bemoaned the fact that one store-bought cucumber in 1801 was just as pricey as a pound of butter.[2] Yet eight years later her fortunes changed again. A return to country life, to her final home at Chawton Cottage, clearly came with one major perk for Jane—condensed in her first eager question about the property: "What sort of a kitchen garden is there?" A rather large one, came the answer, with an orchard, a vegetable patch, and hedgerows too. Soon "a great crop" of everything from plums to peas was back on the Austen family table.

Everyone equated living well with eating "green" throughout the era. In Tobias Smollett's 1771 novel *Humphry Clinker*, a rich country squire enjoys the long-winded boast that "At Brambleton Hall . . . my table is, in a great measure, furnished from my own ground . . . My salads, roots, and pot herbs, my own garden yields in plenty and perfection . . . The same soil affords all the different fruits which England may call her own, so that my dessert is every day fresh gathered from the tree."[3] Every "decent" Englishman "has his garden, which is half his support as well as his delight," wrote the naturalist Gilbert White in 1789, noting how much the nation's "consumption of vegetables has increased" because of it.[4] I prefer the simpler findings of one Monsieur Louis Simond, a French traveler to England in 1810: "Vegetables" to the English, he said, were "like hay to horses."[5]

Enjoyed for their own sake, not just as a filler or adjunct to meat, the English loved to get adventurous with their "garden stuff," dabbling in growing different varieties of old favorites or trying something totally new. Austen writes about the thrill of tasting a weird, red, and

rumpy-looking fruit newly imported from the Americas—
tomatoes. So new, Jane adorably flounders on the spelling,
calling them "tomatas" and insists her sister try them too.
"Have you any tomatas? Fanny [my niece] and I regale
on them every day." In *Northanger Abbey*, Catherine also
thrills over General Tilney's new-fangled "pinery" (a hot-
house for growing the then very posh and exotic pineap-
ple). The general laments that he *only* gets about "one
hundred" pineapples a year—another backhanded brag—
but such were the "inconveniences" of a rich gentleman
in a world where the most fashionable tables were kept as
bountifully garden fresh as possible.

In her simpler way, Austen loved keeping up with the
Tilneys whenever she could, pottering about in her own
kitchen garden at Chawton and getting the "agreeable surprise" of finding the first summer strawberries in the patch
or detecting the first "apricot . . . on one of the trees."
Today, those who have grown anything remotely edible
(even if it's just a pot of parsley on the fire escape) can
relate to Austen's agreeable surprises and fuzzy feelings
for her little plot of earth. "The garden is quite a love,"
she said. But once this lovely "garden stuff" got into her
kitchen, things started to look a little different from what
we might expect today. Austen didn't go wild and crazy with
her vegetable cookery (she didn't mold her boiled spinach
into the pudgy likeness of the Prince Regent, in case you're
worried), but there are a few historical differences in how
Jane approached this edible "English verdure."

Like everything else in Austen's kitchen, plants came with distinct dietary rules—ways to enjoy and eat them most healthfully. Nothing wacky, just the Regency take on traditional plant-eating strategies inherited the world over. Some of them you might recognize, others have been almost forgotten in recent years, *"but as it happens, they are all of them very clever."*

"Very Thoroughly Boiled"

Perhaps the main reason the Regency era developed such a misunderstood veggie reputation was due to its strict views on cooking them. Whereas we might look at a platter of raw, crisp vegetables versus a pot of cooked, soft vegetables and jump to the quick conclusion that the raw option is healthier, people in Austen's era did the opposite. For them, the historic rule of thumb upheld that a cooked vegetable was generally safer than a raw one. Some people even cooked their cucumbers. I personally "eat them stewed," said one Regency parson with dietary pride.[6]

Yet don't chuckle too quickly. Every traditional culture, from Asia to the Americas, has thought along these exact lines. Rather than viewing the vegetable kingdom as one big raw bar to casually nibble through, our ancestors were much more cautious about their "garden stuff." For them, most vegetables were regarded as tricky little foods that needed the magic of cooking to make them more nutritious. Their reasons were twofold, and both equally smart. On the one hand, they knew that starchy

vegetables are always easier to digest once cooked—
heat breaks down and releases the edible energy trapped
inside tough plant tissue. On the other hand, they recognized that many plants in their raw state come with
natural toxins humans should carefully avoid.[7] Given our
modern raw-equals-healthier outlook, we tend to forget
how chemically potent and problematic many raw plant
foods actually are. Legumes especially (peas, beans, lentils)
contain high traces of lectin compounds, natural toxins
that can cause serious gastrointestinal distress when not
cooked properly. Raw lima beans have a chemical that
turns into cyanide in our bodies (yes, as in full-on Agatha
Christie cyanide), and eating just four raw kidney beans is
enough to give you lectin poisoning.[8] Uncooked crucifer-
ous vegetables, such as cabbage, broccoli, and kale (often
added to modern "green" smoothies) contain goitrogenic
chemicals that can interfere with the proper working of
your thyroid. The same goes for raw spinach, okra, egg-
plant, and swiss chard—all containing oxalates and phytates, "anti-nutrients" that can block your body's ability
to absorb essential minerals like calcium, zinc, and iron.

Cooking has always been the easiest way to neutral-
ize these potentially noxious compounds, the safest way
to approach most vegetables, something firmly established throughout most of food history from the Regency
era backward. In *Emma*, anxious Mr. Woodhouse (with
his usual love for jumping to extremes) seems to insist
that anything out of the ground should be cooked "three

times" over—a comic exaggeration even by Regency standards. Because despite the lingering stereotype, Austen and her fellow veggie aficionados didn't overcook their garden stuff down to a pulpy mush. They loved the vibrant color, freshness, and flavor of vegetables and certainly didn't enjoy ruining them with "over-anxious caution." Writing in *The British Housewife* (one of the era's most popular cookbooks), Martha Bradley reminds her readers that spinach only needs a few minutes of gentle cooking before it's ready for the table.[9] Salads were also popular at the time, deemed perfectly acceptable to eat raw and crisp. Notice that the ladies of Longbourn enjoy a "cold" cucumber salad at their luncheon in *Pride and Prejudice*. And yet, cooking most "garden stuff" properly was still viewed as integral to overall health—an outlook we can still embrace with dietary sense today.

In fact, it's now confirmed that many vegetables become *more* nutrient and vitamin rich when a little heat is applied. Tomatoes, for instance, give off more of the antioxidant lycopene when cooked, and carrots release far higher levels of beta-carotene (becoming vitamin A in the body). Cooking also benefits asparagus, breaking down its fibrous cell walls and increasing our ability to absorb its vitamins and ferulic acid. The same goes for mushrooms; we can't fully tap into their unique nutritional value until they're cooked.[10] Steaming things up with a little lively "heat and animation," as they say in *Persuasion*, has its uses.

"He Loved Good Fruit"

We've already explored Jane's relationship with fruit in previous chapters, but it's worth noting how enlightened her views were. At the time, the usual attitude was that fruits (just like vegetables) should be given a thorough cooking before they were safe to eat. Eating raw fruit—eating raw *anything*—had been regarded as risky to health since antiquity (not an unwise prejudice, considering heat was the easiest way to kill unwanted bacteria). You'll notice old-fashioned Mr. Woodhouse only recommends "wholesome" cooked fruit in *Emma*. But as Jane points out, Mr. Woodhouse is a bit behind the times. Since 1747, sailors in the British navy began recognizing the curative power of raw fruit for preventing scurvy[11] (a disease caused by the dietary lack of vitamin C—a heat-sensitive vitamin damaged whenever fruit is cooked). With two brothers in the navy, Jane was evidently aware of this newfound respect for raw fruit, including many references in her novels. Beginning in *Sense and Sensibility* (where Mrs. Jennings and Charlotte happily "stuff" themselves with mulberries straight from the tree) it follows through to *Emma*, where the ladies of Highbury are convinced that strawberries, picked from the ground and popped in the mouth, are decidedly "wholesome"—"the only way of really enjoying them." Cutting-edge claims for 1815, still wonderfully accurate over two hundred years later.

"The Butter, the Celery, the Beet-Root"

On to Austen's next vegetable rule: to the Regency mind, a vegetable wasn't ready for consumption unless it was properly "dressed." Austen speaks of receiving a present of "seacale" (sea kale) in 1817 but defers eating it until the time comes for "dressing it." And just to clarify, this isn't a reference to salad dressing or, for the more young at heart, a weird proclivity for outfitting veggies in Regency costumes (though I commend your spirit and join you in thinking that a Darcy-dressed daikon might certainly be fun). "Dressing" a vegetable for Jane meant serving it with a succulent sauce, usually made with liberal quantities of cream or butter. A butter sauce was "the usual method of dressing vegetables in England," said Carl Moritz, a Swiss visitor in 1782.[12] Later we find Mr. Elton of *Emma* listing "butter" in the same breath alongside "celery" and "beet-root"—the vegetables served at the Cole's dinner party. A "melted butter" sauce is likewise indispensable on Henry Tilney's table in *Northanger Abbey*.

Hardly unique to Regency England, you'll find this vegetable/fat pattern repeating the world over. From the Italian habit of drizzling olive oil generously over every vegetable in sight, to the Indian tradition of serving spinach with large chunks of paneer cheese, to Southern grandmothers dutifully stewing collard greens with lots of bacon, the cross-cultural consensus is pretty solid: vegetables should be eaten with fat.

The best explanation for this was revealed in 2004, when scientists at Iowa State University carried out a now famous experiment. For twelve weeks, college students were given a bowl of salad (with spinach, carrots, and tomatoes) and a range of salad dressings, from fat-free to full-fat dressings, to enjoy it with. Then their blood was tested. Remarkably, though everyone ate the same salad, the students who ate their greens without any fat didn't absorb any of its healthy antioxidants called carotenoids. Brightly colored nutrients found in carrots, tomatoes, and leafy vegetables, carotenoids turn into vitamin A in our bodies. Yet despite *eating* the carotenoids, "essentially no beta-carotene" was absorbed without the aid of fat. Only when a little oil was drizzled over their salad did the nutrient ever get absorbed.[13]

While theoretically understood since the early twentieth century (i.e., that many vitamins are "fat soluble," meaning they need fat to be properly dissolved), it was all too easy to forget during the frenzied fat fears of the 1990s. But I'm afraid munching on dry carrot sticks or eating plain steamed broccoli wouldn't be "very fashionable" to Jane, and neither is it very functional today. You'll get the fiber from the vegetable, but not much else. Instead, follow the historic rule of thumb: if your vegetables have any color at all, those colors mean vitamins, and those vitamins need some sort of fat to wash them down healthfully. Even ditsy Lydia Bennet understands that much. She doesn't "triumphantly" display her luncheon table in *Pride and Prejudice* until she's spent a thoughtful moment "dressing a salad and cucumber."

"Here Is a Nut . . . a Beautiful Glossy Nut"

I'll belabor you with no puns, dear reader, with this brief look on going nuts in Austenworld. Jane doesn't mention nuts very frequently, but when she does, there's a clever insight attached. In *Persuasion*, Louisa and Captain Wentworth try their hand at "gleaning" for hazelnuts in a nearby hedgerow during the novel's "long walk." Austen reminds us that this is happening in autumn—the only time when hazelnuts are naturally found in England's hedgerows. Nuts were only a seasonal indulgence in the Regency era, and oftentimes hard to find when they *were* in season. Harriet talks of enjoying "walnuts" in *Emma* but points out that Mr. Martin had to search "three miles round" to glean her "some." And once people got their hands on nuts, they were the natural tough-nut-to-crack types (buying a bulk-sized bag of already-shelled nuts was a distant luxury). And with all this gleaning and cracking, nobody had the patience to eat more than a handful at a time. Not only is this the way most people ate nuts for most of human history, it's how the majority of health experts still recommend eating them—in small handful-like quantities. While smart on a weight-management front (nuts are deceptively energy dense), raw nuts are also high in phytates, the same "anti-nutrients" present in some vegetables. You don't want to be eating large quantities every day. Save nuts for those occasional, delicious treats, eating about as many as one might reasonably expect while "gleaning" with your friends from Uppercross.

Pickled Cucumbers

Makes 1 large jar

"Tell you father, with Aunt Cass's love and mine,
that the pickled cucumbers are extremely good."
—Austen's letters

Pickling skyrocketed in popularity during Austen's day, with the Regency palate loving the flavor contrast of tart vegetables and cold meat. The Austens had an entire "cucumber garden" at Steventon for keeping a steady supply of pickles on the table.

INGREDIENTS

1 cup water

½ cup distilled white vinegar

2 garlic cloves, peeled and smashed

1 tablespoon sugar

2 teaspoons salt

1 medium-sized cucumber (about 12 ounces)

1 tablespoon chopped fresh dill

1. Put the water, vinegar, garlic, sugar, and salt in a saucepan. Bring to a simmer over high heat, stirring to dissolve sugar and salt. Remove from heat and let cool.

2. While the liquid is cooling, cut the cucumber into thick round slices, about ¼-inch thick. Put into a large mason jar (or any convenient bowl).

3. Add the chopped dill to the cooled liquid, then pour over the cucumbers. Cover the container (with a lid or plastic wrap) and refrigerate for 24 hours to allow the cucumbers to soak up the pickling liquid.

"The cucumber will, I believe, be
a very acceptable present."
—Austen's letters

"I shall now take the liberty of wishing
them health and happiness."

—*Pride and Prejudice*

7

"HEALTH AND HAPPINESS": THE MIND-BODY CONNECTION

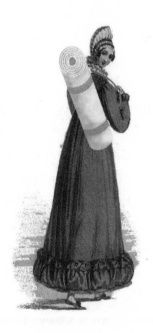

"*Going so soon! This must not be.*" I'm afraid so. Our journey through the health secrets of Austenworld is almost over. But there is one final trip to make before we can all live healthily ever after. Think of it as a sort of pilgrimage—an enlightening climb up the Regency equivalent of a Tibetan monastery. Inside, Jane Austen might not look like your typical Zen master—the requisite cup of green tea being the only earthly connection—but the woman is pretty good at bending mind over matter. According to Jane, all of us have the power to think, feel, and will ourselves to better health—some of the most far-out medical mysteries science has only started deciphering. And Austen has been tapping into the power of the mind for over three centuries: in novels that promote the medicinal magic of happiness, warn us of the biological damage of stress, and remind us that the "mind and body" always function "alike."

"I believe in a true analogy between our bodily frames and our mental." These were some of the last published words Austen wrote, and they prop up her entire health philosophy. As integral as food or exercise, thoughts and feelings were potent things to Jane, healing or harming our bodies depending on how carefully we manage our minds. "I must take care of my mind," says Fanny in *Mansfield Park*—every life in Austenworld literally hinges on it. How accurately that applies to our own stories will soon be explored. So hold on to your wispy straw bonnets, we're about to get "strange, wild," and metaphysical with Jane.

"Glowing and Lovely . . . in Happiness"

Embracing the patriotic spirit of Regency England (England and France were at war for most of Austen's lifetime), let's begin our mind-body lesson by doing the historically respectable thing: blaming the French. The main reason most of us find the whole mind-over-matter concept so "strange" and "wild" today is largely thanks to the seventeeth-century French philosopher René Descartes. Descartes believed that the ethereal emotions of our minds and the physical mechanics of our bodies were two separate entities, arguing that since they functioned independently from each other, they should be studied independently. His theory would largely influence our modern conception of the solid split between mental health and physical health.[1]

Yet Austen never knew to separate the two, living in an age when the mind and body were still intimately linked. "There is nothing of which the physician is more frequently aware, than of the power of the mind," wrote philosopher William Godwin in 1798,[2] around the sametime Jane was writing *Northanger Abbey*. People had been connecting the mind-body dots since (and before) the Roman poet Juvenal penned his pithy motto—*mens sana in corpore sano*—"a sound mind in a sound body." And for Jane, a sound mind naturally meant a happy one.

Given her father's position as a rector in the Church of England, Jane would have grown up hearing the biblical proverb she clearly understood as literal: "a joyful heart is good medicine." Very soon her fictional rector, Mr. Collins, would make the same connection in *Pride and Prejudice*. "As for my fair cousins . . . I shall now take the liberty of wishing them health and happiness." He repeats the sentiment twice, as does Darcy: "accept my best wishes for your health and happiness." It soon becomes very clear that you can't have one without the other in Austenworld.

It's usually shrugged off as just another one of Jane's sentimental plot devices—the way mood so intensely affects the overall health of her characters. On one extreme, Marianne nearly dies of a broken heart over her "violent sorrow" for Willoughby. On another, Anne Elliot comes fully alive the happier she feels, "glowing and lovely" in "very good health and very good looks." Smiles or frowns become such strong predictors of health in Jane's novels, it isn't surprising when the narrator of *Emma* expects us to believe that Jane Fairfax is a physical product of how she feels. Spending most of the novel worried and depressed over her illicit engagement to Frank Churchill, her sickness and sadness, her sickness and sadness, her "troubles" and "ill health" have "the same origin," we are told. Yet when finally "happy" again, Jane Fairfax bounces back to health in only a few short chapters: "Emma had never seen her look so well, so lovely." Gee, *that* was fast, we snicker. These are romantic *fictions*, after all. But they also reflect a core belief of classical medicine.

"Confidence and hope do more good than physic," wrote Galen, the second-century Greek physician, still well respected in the Regency medical community.[3] William Godwin was so much in agreement, he went on to define sadness as "the brother of death. But cheerfulness gives new elasticity to our limbs, and circulation to our juices."[4] Someone who could use a good circulation of her juices is Mrs. Smith, Anne's close friend in *Persuasion*. Though suffering from a crippling illness in dismal living conditions with no money to pay the doctor bills, Mrs. Smith remains remarkably positive and upbeat through-out her trials. She had a "deposition" to "be cheerful . . . neither sickness nor sorrow seemed to have closed her heart or ruined her spirits." It pays off. Her cheerful mind soon becomes a mysterious pathway to her medical cure. Mrs. Smith's "cheerfulness and mental alacrity did not fail her," and she gradually experiences "improvement of health" by the end of the novel.

Putting it in modern terms, Austen was one of the first novelists to promote the power of positive thinking—boldly claiming that "health, good humour, and cheerfulness" are biologically connected. It was her infamous "shove it" to Descartes' splintered medical theory, and it would prove to be, scientifically, centuries ahead of its time. Not until the 1980s would researchers first discover that Descartes was wrong, that there is a direct bridge between the feelings in our heads and the functions of our bodies. Now studied (appropriately) under the massive bridge-looking term of psychoneuroimmunology, scientists have found that our mood matters, particularly to our immune system. Positive emotions like happiness and hope allow our brains to release chemicals that strengthen the immune system, whereas negative thoughts release chemicals that suppress it.[5] In short, happiness makes it easier for your body to both fight illnesses and heal more quickly from them.

As Austen observes in *Pride and Prejudice*, when people are happy, it "displayed itself over their whole bodies." It gives Jane Bennet "a glow . . . of complexion," adds a delightful "lustre" to Lizzie's eyes, and, in *Sense and Sensibility*, makes Mrs. Dashwood look "brilliant" and younger than ever. No wonder Austenites are constantly reminding themselves to be happy. "I will endeavor to banish every painful thought, and think only of what will make me happy." It's the creed of every smart and healthy character, the insistence that no matter what life throws at you—a canceled picnic at Delaford, a conniving Lucy Steele with earth-shattering secrets ("did I mention I'm engaged to Edward?")—you never should lose your "composure of mind."

Elinor does it with extraordinary zeal in *Sense and Sensibility*. Her mental composure is legendary ("So calm! so cheerful!") even in the face of relentless adversity. Others might attempt to thwart her "peace of mind," Lucy Steele *might* let it slip that she's a man-stealing hussy, but Elinor knows how to "govern" her feelings and recovers from the bad news within seconds: "her heart sunk within her" but "she struggled so resolutely against the oppression of her feelings, that her success was speedy." And when Elinor isn't practicing self-composure herself, she's reminding everyone else to do it—"be composed" "pray, pray be composed."

Lines like that tend to make modern readers squirm in their seats. It sounds uncomfortably like Austen is asking us to suppress our true feelings, convincing ourselves that we are happy when we're not. Apparently, Jane's quick answer to therapy is "buck up and shut up." But it's far more clever than that. Characters like Elinor are actually practicing one of the fundamentals of modern psychology: selective attention. It's the common-sense understanding that we can only experience negative emotions when we actively think about them, in the present moment. And since most negative thoughts are the result of either ruminating over past traumas or future worries, we always have the power (right now, right here) *not* to give our attention to them. I'll concede, this doesn't exactly meld with our current therapy culture, with its endless requirements to talk about and analyze our darker emotions, but one of the fathers of modern psychology, William James, was saying it back in the 1890s: "My experience is what I agree to attend to."[6] Every Austen character is endowed with this same mental freedom, the ability to focus on either negative or positive emotions at any given time. "You must learn some of my philosophy," says Lizzie. "Think only of the past as its remembrance gives you pleasure." Austen calls it emotional "courting," choosing your thoughts as wisely as you would choose your marriage partner. In *Emma*, Frank Churchill is reprimanded for choosing wrongly, dwelling on painful memories for longer than necessary: "How you can bear such recollections, is astonishing to me!—They *will* sometimes obtrude—but how you can court them!"

Elinor and Marianne: A Case Study

Throughout *Sense and Sensibility*, Austen asks us to consider the important question: Is it better to frequently release our "sorrows" (like Marianne) or try to "subdue" them (like Elinor). After her breakup with Willoughby, Marianne clearly thinks it's better to scream into the proverbial pillow. "Without any desire of command over herself," she lets it rip. "I must feel—I must be wretched." Many people would still agree: that releasing our anger and frustrations makes us feel better. Better than bottling them up, right? Surprisingly, no. Researchers at Iowa State University found that when people are angry, giving them the opportunity to "vent" their anger (by ruminating over the problem and punching something) actually makes them feel *more* aggressive, negative, and angrier than people who don't vent.[7] A few exhausting pillows screams later and Marianne eventually reaches the same conclusion, telling Elinor: "I saw that my own feelings had prepared my sufferings, and that my want of fortitude under them had almost led me to the grave." "I compare [my conduct] with what it ought to have been; I compare it with yours."

"Courting" negative thoughts is always a dangerous business in Jane's novels. It won't just "ruin your happiness," it will wreck your health. Which brings us to the biggest health horror of Austenworld: stress.

"My Poor Nerves"

Stress in Austenworld? Surely not. "What calm lives they had, those people!" sniffed Winston Churchill, not exactly enthralled by the action-packed sequence of *Pride of Prejudice*.[8] No explosions, no battle scenes, no terrorists' threats—what could Austenites possibly be stressed out about? Their tea not being hot enough? It's a stereotype that has ammoed Jane's critics since the very beginning. "I should hardly like to live with her ladies and gentlemen in their elegant but confined houses," yawned Charlotte Brontë in 1848.[9] Much too "common-place" and "neat" for her wilder passions. Um, pardon me, are we all reading the same books here? Because stress is not only very much present in Austenworld, it's practically an epidemic.

Granted, Jane never uses the word "stress" like we use it today—stress wasn't coined as a biological condition until the 1930s—but she certainly knew it by other names. A multitude of Regency terms like "flutterings," "fidgets," "agitations," "vexations," and, above all, "nerves" are the historical equivalents to what we would now recognize as physiological stress. They fizz up in Jane's novels with vengeance. Once you take off the rose-tinted spectacles (I'm looking at you, Charlotte) you'll find Austenworld is seething with some of the most intensely stressful scenarios any of us will ever face: Your son falls from a tree, nearly paralyzing himself (*Persuasion*). Your home may be handed over to a distant relative at any moment (*Pride and Prejudice*). Your once substantial income drops to near poverty levels overnight (*Sense and Sensibility*). Small wonder many Austen characters find it difficult to cope with the stress—Mrs. Bennet most iconically. The constant frazzle of getting five daughters married before her husband kicks the bucket (when Mr. Collins, in turn, will kick "herself and her daughters out of the house") is too much for her "poor nerves" to bear. She eventually snaps, becoming bedridden by the financial anxiety: "Mrs. Bennet was really in a most pitiable state." "I am frightened out of my wits," she says, "and have such tremblings, such flutterings, all over me, such spasms in my side, and pains in my head, and such beatings at heart, that I can get no rest by night nor by day." If that's not an accurate depiction of extreme stress in action, I don't know what is!

Yet the idea that this was acceptable—nay, encouraged—behavior was rampant throughout the late eighteenth century. Ever since Jane was young, stress itself was viewed as the right and prerogative of the rich and well-off. The more stress you felt, the more you demonstrated to the world how truly delicate and sensitive your wealthy, softly pampered body actually was. The common catchword for this was having a heightened *sensibility*—one of the most fashionable afflictions in England at the time.[10] Mainly affecting the "nerves," a Regency woman who caught the sensibility bug "disdains to be strong minded," wrote a cultural observer in 1799, "she trembles at every breeze, faints at every peril and yields to every assailant."[11] Austen knew real-life strutters of this sensibility, writing about one acquaintance who rather enjoys "her spasms and nervousness and the consequence they give her." It's the same "sensibility" Marianne wallows in throughout the novel that bears its name, "feeding and encouraging" her anxiety "as a duty." Readers of the era would have found nothing out of the ordinary in Marianne's high-strung embrace of stress. What's extraordinary is Jane's response to it.

"Do Not Give Way to Such Gloomy Thoughts"

Rather than taking the normal Regency stance, viewing stress as an innocent indulgence of the upper classes—letting Marianne enjoy her sensibility in peace or allowing Mrs. Bennet her "nervous" tantrum in bed—Jane makes it repeatedly clear that stress is "not to be trifled with." It's no random pattern that stress sickens, weakens, and incapacitates more bodies in her novels than anything else. Jane took stress seriously. If you doubt it, try getting chronically stressed out in Austenworld. She'll usually threaten you with death for doing so.

Marianne is the classic example. After being dumped by Willoughby, she stews for weeks in "silent agony" "till her heart was so heavy that no further sadness could be gained; and this nourishment of grief was every day applied." Later, "the severity and danger" of her deadly illness is directly attributed to her "many weeks of previous" emotional stress, "which Marianne's disappointment had brought on." Then again, she's just one of many stress-induced sufferers. Take Jane Fairfax in *Emma*, for example. Anxiety-ridden throughout most of the novel, the stress of constantly hiding her engagement to Frank Churchill soon manifests in "severe headaches and a nervous fever . . . her health seemed for the moment completely deranged." Elsewhere in the novel, Mrs. Churchill (Frank's aunt) is one of those remarkably rare characters to actually die in the course of an Austen novel. What's kills her off? Stress. "Her nerves were under continual irritation and suffering." Mrs. Bennet gets a sort of deathbed warning too. Being constantly "in the fidgets," suffering from chronic fears that her husband will die (leaving her homeless), will probably have the reverse effect in the end. As the far calmer Mr. Bennet wryly portends, "My dear, do not give way to such gloomy thoughts . . . Let us flatter ourselves that *I* may be the survivor."

Even by today's standards, Jane's death-by-stress plotlines seem pretty intense, more often chalked up to romantic exaggeration than medical sense. Many people still regard stress with Regency laxness, viewing it as an inevitable and normal part of life. But since the 1950s, science has been playing catch-up with Jane, gradually defining the seriousness of stress in almost identical ways:

- We now know that stress should only be a quick, short-term sensation. Many animals benefit from the involuntary stress reaction. Its primary purpose has been to keep us and our ancestors alive during life-threatening situations—stopping normal body functions and diverting all energy into the things (heart, brain, limbs) that help us quickly avoid or surmount the danger. To use a period example, let's just say you'd feel more like running or fighting, not casually using the restroom, when being charged by Napoleon's infantry at the Battle of Waterloo. When stress, however, is allowed to linger—when we replay those life battles in our brains or worry about other battles in the future—our normal body functions are given the chronic cold shoulder. Crucial biological processes like healing, cell growth, proper digestion, metabolism, and weight management are all put on "minimal-priority mode" when stress is activated.[12] Austen was very wary of this sort of long term stress. Her healthiest characters are always trying to limit the time-frame of their stress response—to be "only vexed for a moment," not for days or weeks. A stressful thought might be "involuntary," says Elinor, but "I will not encourage it." Left in romantic limbo by Mr. Bingley in *Pride and Prejudice*, Jane Bennet has every right to be chronically stressed too, but "her good sense" soon prevails, helping her "check the indulgence of those regrets which must have been injurious to her own health."

The real "injurious" nature of stress is how much it weakens our immune system (maintaining a healthy immune system being another "non-essential" when you're running from a Napoleonic cannon). Chronic stress dramatically reduces our ability to fight everything from the common cold to cancer, impeding natural repair processes that defend us against viruses, tumors, and inflammation.[13] An astounding 75 to 90 percent of all doctor's visits are now estimated to be stress and inflammation related.[14] Over two hundred years ago, Austen was reflecting these statistics with staggering accuracy. Most illnesses in Austenworld have a corresponding "nervous" component. Emma recognizes "a nervous part to her complaint" when her friend Harriet suffers from a "severe cold" and sore throat. Coincidentally, Harriet has just spent the past few weeks in a constant emotional "flutter" over Mr. Elton. In *Mansfield Park*, the stressful nugget of news that Maria has run off with Henry is enough to derail Fanny's immune system: "She passed only from feelings of sickness to shudderings of horror; and from hot fits of fever to cold." One of the last characters Austen created, Arthur Parker in *Sanditon* (a man with more illnesses than you can count) has a hunch that they all point back to stress. "I am very nervous," he says. "To say the truth, nerves are the worst part of my complaints in *my* opinion."

But the injury of stress goes even deeper than that, damaging our bodies on a genetic level. The ends of our tightly wound chromosomes (capped by a protective telomere—the genetic equivalent to the hard tip on a shoelace string) are particularly sensitive to stress.

While telomeres naturally wear down over time, gradually frazzling our cells and thus aging our bodies, stress can dramatically accelerate the process. People who live under chronic stress have shorter telomeres that sometimes look ten years older than people with less stress in their lives.[15] Again, Austen doesn't miss a biological beat. The characters who experience the most intense stress in her books look literally frazzled and aged beyond their years—Mr. Woodhouse in *Emma*, for instance. "He was a nervous man" with a long-running relationship with stress. There is "no rest for his . . . nerves," and he looks "a much older man" than he actually is. Yet Marianne proves an even bigger warning on the aging effects of stress. Starting the novel a vibrantly "beautiful girl," her later Willoughby-induced stress takes its physical toll. Stress "affected . . . every feature," giving her a "hollow eye" and "sickly skin." Even lovable Edward and Mrs. Jennings can't help but notice she's "an altered creature." Her less-than-lovable brother-in-law is a bit blunter than that: "Poor Marianne . . . You would not it think perhaps, but [she] was remarkably handsome a few months ago; quite as handsome as Elinor.—Now you see it is all gone."

If Austen's own life imitated her art, it's easy to explain why she was so interested in writing about stress and its damaging effects. It was a personal fight. Her surviving letters reveal a woman who was often tempted to indulge in chronic stress: in anger, in money worries, and the endless frustrations of being an intelligent, independent woman in a world which maddeningly limited her freedom. Her biographer David Nokes would go on to argue that Austen chose the alias "Mrs. Ashton Dennis" for writing irritated letters to her publishers just so she could sign it with the clever hint, "I am Gentlemen &c &c MAD."[16]

We don't know how MAD or stressed Austen allowed herself to get, but we do know how greatly she admired the mental composure of her sister Cassandra—a real Elinor and calmer role model throughout Jane's life. Cassandra was no stranger to stress herself—her fiancé died in a heartbreaking incident when she was in her early twenties—but the way Cassandra bravely dealt with the grief ("with a degree of resolution") installed her in Jane's respect forever. With a "temper always under command,"[17] Cassandra must have taught Jane little secrets for managing her own stress, as Austen would soon fill her novels with them. There are numerous, brilliant ways to de-stress in Austenworld, and whether we have Jane or Cassandra to thank for these strategies is a moot point. The point is they work. They obviously worked for Jane and they still work today. So please take Mrs. Bennet's advice and "have a little compassion" on your "poor nerves . . ."

1. "I Will Be Mistress of Myself"

Interestingly, the most stressed-out minds in Austenworld share one thing in common: a lack of control. Pick any anxious character—Mr. Woodhouse, Mrs. Bennet, Mary Musgrove, Jane Fairfax, Marianne—their individual stress always stems from not feeling in control: of either their money, their houses, their love lives, their husbands, their children, their bodies, or their futures. Austen lays out her psychological theory again and again. One's mental comfort (or chaos) primarily depends on feeling "under command" of the situation. As Emma reminds Frank Churchill, once he calms down after a grumpy snap: "You are comfortable [now] because you are under command . . . You had, somehow or other, broken bounds yesterday, and run away from your own management."

Austen would have to wait a few years for that theory to be proven, but proven it was. Throughout the late twentieth century, one of Britain's longest-running research projects, called the Whitehall Study, revealed the powerful benefits of feeling in control. Tracking the long-term health of over twenty-eight thousand workers in the British Civil Service, it found something that defies the usual workplace stereotype. People higher up in the office hierarchy—bosses, superiors, people who had *more* control in their jobs—actually had *less* stress, less disease, and longer lifespans than their subordinates (despite receiving the same medical care). Even with more workplace responsibility, feeling able to confidently manage daily situations acted like a permanent stress reducer.[18]

Putting this into practice, you might want to start thinking like a boss, a Regency boss. Lizzie does so in

Pride and Prejudice. When confronted with the daunting task of meeting Lady Catherine (the biggest boss in Austenworld), Lizzie puffs up her self-confidence, believing she is "quite equal" to the job. She, therefore, walks calmly up to Lady Catherine's imposing house. Her tremulous companions, not so much: "When they ascended the steps to the hall, Maria's alarm was every moment increasing, and even Sir William did not look perfectly calm." But "Elizabeth's courage did not fail her." While the others were "frightened almost out of [their] senses . . . Elizabeth found herself quite equal to the scene."

Feeling "equal" to the Lady Catherines of life—feeling you can handle an unexpected workload, a financial curveball, a family argument, or, in my case, a publishing deadline—is crucial to keeping stress at bay. When Louisa falls off the sea wall at Lyme in *Persuasion*, dangerously concussing her head on the cobbles, Anne is the only one who keeps "her senses," the only one to remember the obvious next best step when a bonneted head comes crashing down onto the pavement: "A surgeon . . . a surgeon this instant." None of us can control how often we are, as Austen would say, "knocked about" by life, but we *can* control our response to it. In *Sense and Sensibility*, Elinor constantly chooses calm, finding immense strength in simply remembering she has the power to choose it: "I *will* be calm; I will be mistress of myself." As Austen knew, there's always that crucial moment between the stressor and our reaction to it. And, if nothing else, that one moment is entirely within our control. "Between stimulus and response there is a space," goes the mindfulness mantra often attributed to Holocaust survivor Viktor Frankl. "In that space is our power to choose our response. In our response lies our growth and freedom."

2. "Laugh as Much as You Choose"

Laughter was always integral to Austen's life. The earliest stories to plop from her pen as a teenager were comedies with slapstick plotlines crafted to elicit a well-timed chuckle. Studying these early texts, Virginia Woolf once asked the important rhetorical question: "What is this note which never merges in the rest, which sounds distinctly and penetratingly all through?" Easy. "It is the sound of laughter."[19] It echoes in Austen's personal letters to her sister, with witty jokes dolloped throughout, and rings loud in *Pride and Prejudice*. Lizzie is always ready for a good laugh, making her the self-proclaimed "happiest creature in the world"—and certainly the happiest heroine. "I dearly love a laugh . . . Follies and nonsense, whims and inconsistencies, do divert me, I own, and I laugh at them whenever I can." Laughter is both an emotional shield and sword to Lizzie, helping her to lighten awkward situations, painful rejections (oh, like being called only "tolerable" by Darcy), and most importantly, stressful situations. "It was necessary to laugh, when she would rather have cried." Lizzie's laugh-away-the-blues reflex is such a well-known family fact, when Jane Bennet spends a few sad months pining over Mr. Bingley, her Aunt Gardiner flatly admits that Lizzie would have dealt with the stressful situation better: "It had better have happened to *you*, Lizzie; you would have laughed yourself out of it sooner."

In 1976, a magazine editor named Norman Cousins famously demonstrated just how far we can laugh ourselves out of negative situations. Diagnosed with a painful, paralyzing disease of the joints and given a one-in-five-hundred chance of recovery, Cousins checked himself out of the hospital to find out if laughter is truly the best medicine. Instead of pain medication, he dosed up on television comedies and humorous literature, soon making "the joyous discovery that ten minutes of genuine belly laughter had an anesthetic effect and would give me at least two hours of pain-free sleep." In weeks to come, Cousins experienced a rapid remission of all debilitating symptoms in his joints and was soon jogging on the beach.[20] A research hub at UCLA now bears his name: The Norman Cousins Center for Psychoneuroimmunology.

Proven to lower blood pressure and reduce stress, even smiling is powerful. Since infancy our brains have been hardwired to associate the act of smiling as an immediate pathway to pleasure. As our cheeks go up, so do our moods (instantly releasing a happy cocktail of pleasurable brain chemicals). This cheek-to-brain connection is so strong, smiling will work as a mood booster even if you aren't in a particularly smiley mood.[21] It works like a charm for Elinor in *Sense and Sensibility*. Told that the man of her dreams is already taken (by the woman of her nightmares, Lucy Steele), Elinor keeps calm and carries on with the help of a fake smile, "a smile" which relieves "very agitated feelings."

"Inhale a Breeze of Mental Strength"

Don't forget to follow your nose when it comes to reducing stress. In Austenworld, it will usually lead to a whiff of lavender. Inhaling the scent of lavender was thought particularly helpful in Jane's day: for calming nerves or soothing aching heads. Smelling lavender is the only thing that quiets Marianne after her stressful encounter with Willoughby at the ball (in the arms of another woman!). Catherine also turns to lavender when approached by the "greatly agitated" Eleanor—she "obliged her to be seated, rubbed [Eleanor's] temples with lavender-water, and hung over her with affectionate solicitude." And just so we're clear, this isn't the wimpy "smelling bottle" routine beloved by the swoon-happy Victorians. Lavender is truly powerful stuff. It contains brain-soothing chemicals so strong, we can literally absorb them through sniffing. Inhalation is one of the best ways to get drugs quickly to the brain and bloodstream (can anyone say cocaine?), and smelling lavender is one of nature's quickest chill pills. It reduces anxiety, calms racing hearts, and has even been shown to reduce the pain and severity of migraine headaches.[22] Like Catherine does in *Northanger Abbey*, rubbing a few drops of "lavender water" on your temples is still one of the best ways to experience lavender's soothing power. (See recipe at the end of the chapter.)

3. "It Is Such a Happiness When Good People Get Together"

Jane's novels aren't too far removed from a modern sitcom. "Somebody is always going or coming," turning up at the back door, popping in for a quick chat, inviting you on a walk, squeezing you for a juicy bit of gossip, a cup of tea, an invite to a ball, and an "oh, why yes. I'd *love* to stay for supper too!" All totally normal in Austenworld, its tight-knit communities are some of the tightest in English literature—a place where keeping this "company" routine going strong is a veritable bragging right. In *Pride and Prejudice*, one of Mrs. Bennet's crowning glories is her circle of "four-and-twenty families" she depends on to pop over at any time—a routine which helps to alleviate her stress-prone mind, bringing her daily "solace." A frequent popper-inner himself, Sir John sums it up best in the 2008 remake of *Sense and Sensibility*, "Company, company, where would we be without company?"[23] An interesting question science has started unraveling the answer to.

Since the 1950s, researchers have noticed that people who live in close-knit communities, who keep "company" like Austenites, tend to live longer, healthier lives. The most legendary example of this occurred in a small Pennsylvanian town called Roseto, the closest science has come to observing Regency "society" in action. The residents of Roseto didn't eat, drink, work, or exercise any differently than their surrounding neighbors (in fact, they ate worse and smoked heavily), and yet, Roseto seemed like the fountain of youth. Rosetans lived longer and had much lower rates of heart disease than people in surrounding towns. Researchers spent years working out the riddle before coming to one conclusion: the only real difference about the Roseto lifestyle was something Jane would call "visiting." Rosetans spent more time with each other, dropping by for frequent visits, attending the same church, celebrating the same festivals, joining the same social clubs. It all acted like a buffer against daily life stress and depression. The community pulled together during hard times and worked out their problems across kitchen tables. Nobody spent, or was allowed to spend, too much time alone.[24]

Wickham mirrors the exact sentiment in *Pride and Prejudice*: "Society, I own, is necessary to me . . . my spirits will not bear solitude"—perhaps the only truthful thing to come out of his slippery mouth. People need people to stay mentally healthy. The nineteenth-century French sociologist Émile Durkheim was one of the first to officially recognize the mental dangers and health risks of "anomie"—the breakdown of social norms and close community ties.[25] Decades before, Austen was also warning against shunning "company" and being too often alone. Marianne's frequent

THE JANE AUSTEN DIET

habit for taking "solitary walks" doesn't help relieve her near-suicidal sorrows over Willoughby, they increase them, producing "effusions of sorrow as lively as ever." Also prone to depression, Colonel Brandon starts mentally spiraling after spending too "many hours of each day" "entirely alone"—a condition "favourable for the admission of every melancholy idea." Company-loving Sir John sees all this and, no wonder, fears only one thing in his own life: "the dread of being alone."

But that's what friends are for in Austenworld. Jane speaks of the medicinal "balm" of friendship—a potent soother of life stress. "The comfort of such a friend at that moment . . . how grateful was it felt!—a companion whose judgement would guide, whose attendance must relieve, and whose friendship might soothe her!" Lizzie finds emotional "relief" in chatting with Charlotte Lucas, Emma finds "refreshment" in visiting longtime chum Mrs. Weston. And take note: these aren't "friends" on a screen, but the "real, honest, old-fashioned" sort of friends. Whether it's one, two, or "four-and-twenty"—connecting more regularly with your own "idea of good company" will support your mental strength and might just save your life.

4. "An Interval of Meditation"

Sometimes, Austen heroines have to go off the mental grid, to process those shocking "articles of news" that seem to pummel them daily. You know, the typical "your sister just ran off with a proven sex offender," "your creepy preacher just made a pass at you," "the gorgeous man you rejected eight years ago just moved back to the neighborhood and now he's bitter." Those sorts of things: *"Nothing very bad. The fate of thousands."* Every life is guaranteed its fair share of mental shake-ups. And when they come, heroines throughout Austenworld calm back down with the Regency version of "meditation."

Emma, Anne, Elinor, and Lizzie all practice it—frequently needing mental "take fives"—quick retreats to somewhere quiet where their brains can ask a few therapeutic questions: what the heck just happened, how do I feel about it, and how am I going to respond? "An interval of mediation . . . was the best corrective." A few minutes of quiet "solitude" in her bedroom allows Lizzie to wrap her mind around the weirdness of Charlotte marrying Mr. Collins. Emma likewise depends on "separating" herself, now and then, for the "relief of quiet reflection," especially after Mr. Elton's gross proposal. Sure, these "meditations" might look a bit amateurish for those of us accustomed to viewing meditation as a complicated, crossed-legged combo of heavy breathing, brass bells, and deep chants. But Austen never knew meditation in those Eastern-mystic terms. For her, the real magic of mediation lay in simply experiencing the power of "delightful quiet."

Silence, stillness, quiet. Most of us don't fully experience it today until we're fast asleep, but Austen knew that being cognitively silent, from time to time, was essential to a healthy mind. "The quietness of it does me good," she wrote her sister in 1813, describing her enjoyment of a few moments of "snug" solitude with "the front drawing room all to myself." Her novels are arranged accordingly. Nobody functions well without frequent doses of "suitable quietness." In *Emma*, Jane Fairfax automatically correlates her decline in mental health to the absence of silence in her life: "I have never known the blessing of one tranquil hour." Fanny Price can relate. The "incessant noise" and clamor of her family's house in Portsmouth gives Fanny an "aching head," both literal and mental. She longs, "above all," for "the peace and tranquility" of Mansfield Park. In fact, one of the overarching themes in *Mansfield Park* is the pursuit of this quiet, restorative peace. As Lionel Trilling wrote in his famous preface to the novel, *"Mansfield Park* . . . discovers in principal the path to the wholeness of the self which is peace."

Humans have long understood that being constantly surrounded by noise has a negative effect on our minds. Even the word *noise* (from Latin *nausea*) means a form of "sickness." Quietness is a primal need. Our brains are built to require occasional periods of silence to reboot themselves, like computers: downloading, processing, and organizing data more efficiently during quiet moments, even growing more brain cells to smarten our response to the new information.[26] It's no fluke that people often get their best ideas in the "quiet" of a shower, bath, or bed. And it's why Austen heroines, like Anne in *Persuasion*, eagerly seek out quiet times for when they have important "feelings" to "investigate." Silence allows us to process our emotions and solve problems much more successfully.

Yet despite living in the far quieter world of Regency England, Austen knew that silence was a "luxury" you have to consciously remind yourself to enjoy. "Let us have the luxury of silence," says Fanny. So take a short mental holiday on a regular basis, quietly "sitting in unwearied contemplation" for a few minutes without the sound of a phone, TV, radio, or podcast. Just two minutes of silence has been found to be more mentally recharging than listening to relaxing music.[27] In Austenworld, sometimes the best thing to do, hear, or say is absolutely nothing at all. Such is the healthy art of "important nothings" Mrs. Norris in *Mansfield Park* has yet to discover: "Mrs. Norris . . . was now trying to be in a bustle without having anything to bustle about, and labouring to be important where nothing was wanted but tranquility and silence."

5. "A Fine, Stout, Healthy Love"

I'd earn myself a proper Regency tar-and-feathering if I ignored the most potent mental medicine in Jane's arsenal: the one thing pursued in her books more than any other, what holds Austen's entire universe together and makes us, three centuries later, keep coming back for more—*"So much love . . . awaited her there."*

Austen realized that being human automatically binds us in a "contract" with others. Like the subtle give-and-take motions of a ballroom dance, life makes us enter "into a contract of mutual agreeableness" with other humans, "and all our agreeableness belongs solely to each other for that time." In biological terms: we need to feel and give love to stay mentally healthy. It's hardwired in our hormones. Feeling emotionally connected with others releases the "bonding" hormone oxytocin—a chemical crucial for lowering stress and daily anxiety—usually responsible for that cloud-nine feeling of falling in love. And you don't need your own Darcy to experience it.

As far as Jane is concerned, romance isn't always the steadiest source of these "healthy love" connections. As Elinor reminds Marianne after being jilted by Willoughby: "Have you no comforts? no friends? Is your loss such as leaves no opening for consolation?" Very true. Oxytocin can be triggered *anytime* we satisfy that emotional "contract" with others: hugging a friend, admiring a newborn baby, or giving a hot meal to the homeless. This was vital to someone like Austen, who never married, and perhaps explains why she provides so many alternatives to experiencing love in her novels. Sister to sister, parent to child, friend to friend. These human contracts are so strong, even feeling love for faceless strangers is a powerful shield against stress and depression. Now a global movement, writing love letters to anonymous strangers (with actual pen and paper, Regency style), then leaving them in public places for anyone to find, has had tremendous impacts on the mental health of thousands.[28] I once found one of these tokens of kindness on a walk a few years ago—just seven secret words, but it was life changing. Showing kindness, love, and compassion to others (having "tenderness of heart," as Jane would say) works such therapeutic magic because it forces us to turn outward, away from our inward stress and personal pain, and back to what really matters. Whatever her matchmaking faults, Emma has at least figured that much out. After she and Harriet visit and feed "a poor sick family" in the village (the Regency equivalent of working in a soup kitchen), Emma comes away far happier and with mental priorities properly sorted: "These are the sights, Harriet, to do one good. How trifling they make everything else appear!"

You might not get the nuances of love always right (Emma hardly does!) but you can't go far wrong with it, either. Our brains and bodies are always "the better for such well-timed kindness." I can't help but find it all wonderfully satisfying, like cracking a good riddle with Emma and Harriet—this love, this one thing which has kept the body of Austen's work alive, fresh and incandescently vibrant as the day she wrote it, can work the same magic in our own bodies today. So we'll take Austen's cue and end with the words she used in one of her last love letters to the world . . .

Everything of Love and Kindness, proper and
improper, must now suffice,
Yours very affectionately, J. Austen.

Lavender Water

Makes 1 cup

"Catherine . . . obliged her to be seated, rubbed her temples with lavender-water, and hung over her with affectionate solicitude."
—*Northanger Abbey*

Lovely for spritzing on pillows or freshly ironed linens, lavender water could either have been bought from a Regency perfumer (Austen mentions procuring "Steele's Lavender Water" for a friend) or made much more inexpensively at home.

INGREDIENTS

1 cup distilled water
1 tablespoon vodka
(or rubbing alcohol)

10 drops pure lavender essential oil

1. Find yourself a willing and elegant "lavender water" container (anything from an old perfume bottle to a spray or spritz bottle).

2. Use a funnel to help pour the water, vodka, and lavender oil into your container. The alcohol is needed to emulsify the ingredients and preserve the freshness of the lavender water.

3. Top with the lid and shake to combine. Made with distilled water, lavender water will stay fresh for a couple of months.

"Full many a flower is born to blush unseen, and waste its fragrance on the desert air."
—*Emma*

EPILOGUE:

"BEHOLD ME IMMORTAL"

It's not often any of us can say that we have a one-up advantage on the inimitable Jane Austen—usually the most clever and witty woman in the room, regardless of century. But the poignant irony of Jane's own "picture of health" is that it was missing one last puzzle piece that we now have in abundance: modern medicine. It's almost certain that a simple round of prescription drugs, antibiotics, or surgeries would have cured her of the mysterious "illness" that manifested in 1816 and worsened throughout the next year. No one really knows what this "illness" was—though recent theories range from cancer to arsenic poisoning—but without recourse to the modern science she so often paralleled in her novels, Jane died in her literary prime at forty-one years old. Far too young, even by Regency standards: her mother lived well into her eighties, her siblings likewise had longevities stretching into their seventies, eighties, even nineties.

And yet, Jane's life and legacy is full of similar ironies. She turned down marriage and a rich, comfortable home for herself, yet gives it to every heroine as the highest happily ever after. She was denied romance by fate, but wrote the greatest romances the world has ever seen. And in the same paradoxical way, her legacy and writings on health are just as exquisitely ironic. That Jane didn't get to experience the full "life and vigour" she gave so generously to her heroines makes her embrace of health even more meaningful, not less. It ultimately proves how brilliantly advanced and illuminated her thinking was for the time, even within the body she was fated to inhabit at the turn of the nineteenth century—a shadowy age full of medical misunderstandings and biological guesswork.

It is, perhaps, why Austen wanted us to look beyond the struggles of her personal life and focus more on the better life and happiness she worked so hard to accurately display in her fiction. "Behold me immortal"—these were some of the last words Jane wrote before she died—a final, heartfelt plea for us to remember her by the timeless gifts she gave to us and her characters, not by what she was personally denied herself. After all, nobody gives up on an Austen-style chance at love and romance just because its creator lived without it. And neither should we abandon Austen's wonderful "picture of health" just because it took three centuries (and the help of modern medicine) to become complete. Appropriately, Jane didn't give up on health either, even nearing the end.

In those final months, she planned to write about health more than ever. The fragments of her final novel, *Sanditon* (set in a seaside spa town), reveal a developing theme of what true health means and how to properly cherish it. We can only guess how many more thoughtful health strategies Austen would have left us in *Sanditon*—whether through eating, exercise, or mental management. We do know, however, that Jane took a dose of her own medicine. Despite often debilitating pain and weakness, Austen stayed remarkably energetic, walking regularly, eating enough, and looking for happiness even in her darkest hour. There's little doubt that doing so delayed the worst stage of her illness for as long as possible, even giving her a brief remission from its symptoms in 1817. It was her final clasp to a philosophy that supported her throughout her brief, though exceptional, life. Wise and real and just as applicable today, it's Jane's firm belief that whatever our personal health struggles or weaknesses, we must always (and only) do our best with what we've been given. And so Austen leaves us with the one simple, truly immortal and universal advice any of us will ever need: "We must think the best, and hope the best, and do the best."

NOTES

In an effort to avoid cluttering the text with superfluous citations, all quotes from either Jane Austen's novels, personal letters, or miscellaneous writings were sourced from the following:

Jane Austen, *Sense and Sensibility* (reprint; London: Penguin, 2003).

Jane Austen, *Pride and Prejudice* (reprint; London: Penguin, 2014).

Jane Austen, *Mansfield Park* (reprint; London: Penguin, 2014).

Jane Austen, *Emma* (reprint; London: Penguin, 2015).

Jane Austen, *Persuasion* (reprint; London: Penguin, 2003).

Jane Austen, *Northanger Abbey* (reprint; London: Penguin, 2003).

Jane Austen, *Lady Susan; The Watsons; Sanditon* (reprint; London: Penguin, 1974).

Deirdre Le Faye, ed., *Jane Austen's Letters*, 4th ed. (Oxford: OUP, 2011).

1. UNIVERSAL TRUTHS

1. Deirdre Le Faye, *Jane Austen: A Family Record*, 2nd ed. (Cambridge: Cambridge University Press), 221.

2. J. A. Cattarin et al., "Body Image, Mood, and Televised Images of Attractiveness: The Role of Social Comparison," *Journal of Social and Clinical Psychology* 19 (2000): 220–39.

3. Roy Porter, *Flesh in the Age of Reason: The Modern Foundations of Body and Soul* (New York: Norton, 2003), 241.

NOTES

4. Harriet Brown, *Body of Truth: How Science, History, and Culture Drive Our Obsession with Weight—And What We Can Do About It* (Boston: Da Capo, 2015), 157.

5. Hillel Schwartz, *Never Satisfied: A Cultural History of Diets, Fantasies, and Fat* (New York: Free Press, 1986).

6. Sander L. Gilman, *Diets and Dieting: A Cultural Encyclopedia* (New York: Routledge, 2008), 35; "Lord Byron: The Celebrity Diet Icon" by Louise Foxcroft, *BBC News*, January 3, 2012. Available at http://www.bbc.com/news/magazine-16351761.

7. A foundation of classical medicine, this nature-reliant health theory commonly revolved around the "non-naturals"—environmental factors that humans could easily balance for better health. Usually six in total, the non-naturals were defined by eighteenth-century doctor George Cheyne as "1. The Air we breathe in. 2. Our Meat and Drink. 3. Our Sleep and Watching. 4. Our Exercise and Rest. 5. Our Evacuations and their Obstructions. 6. The Passions of our Minds." Porter, *Flesh in the Age of Reason*, 232.

8. "Glutathione: The Mother of All Antioxidants" by Mark Hyman, *Huffington Post*, June 10, 2010. Available at https://www.huffingtonpost.com/dr-mark-hyman/glutathione-the-mother-of_b_530494.html.

9. L. Cai et al., "Purification, Preliminary Characterization and Hepatoprotective Effects of Polysaccharides from Dandelion Root," *Molecules* 22 (2017): 1409; "7 Ways Dandelion Tea Could Be Good for You" by Anna Schaefer, *Healthline*, September 26, 2017. Available at https://www.healthline.com/health/ways-dandelion-tea-could-be-good-for-your#1.

2. "OUR DEVOURING PLAN"

1. Maggie Lane, *Jane Austen and Food* (London: Hambledon, 1995), 81.

2. Traci Mann, *Secrets from the Eating Lab: The Science of Weight Loss, the Myth of Willpower, and Why You Should Never Diet Again* (New York: Harper Wave, 2015), 132–33.

NOTES

3. A 2011 study showed that your brain during prolonged periods of hunger literally begins to consume itself (specifically in the hypothalamus region), only intensifying the onslaught of hunger signals. And who among us can argue with a cannibalistic brain? S. Kaushik et al., "Autophagy in Hypothalamic AgRP Neurons Regulates Food Intake and Energy Balance," *Cell Metabolism* 14 (2011): 173–83.

4. Lane, *Jane Austen and Food*, 78; Leslie A. Marchand ed., *Lord Byron: Selected Letters and Journals* (Cambridge: Harvard University Press, 1982), 62.

5. Gina Kolata, *Rethinking Thin: The New Science of Weight Loss—and the Myths and Realities of Dieting* (New York: Farrar, Straus and Giroux, 2007), 107–109; Ancel Keys et al., *The Biology of Human Starvation*, 2 vols. (Minneapolis: University of Minnesota Press, 1950), 853.

6. Lucy Worsley, *If Walls Could Talk: An Intimate History of the Home* (New York: Walker and Company, 2011), 250.

7. J. E. Painter, "How Visibility and Convenience Influence Candy Consumption," *Appetite* 38 (2002): 237–38.

8. Imagery from a 1793 satirical cartoon entitled "French Happiness/English Misery." Kirstin Olsen, *Daily Life in 18th-Century England* (Westport, CT: Greenwood Press, 1999), 236.

9. Carolly Erickson, *Our Tempestuous Day: A History of Regency England* (New York: William Morrow, 1986), 221.

10. Lane, *Jane Austen and Food*, 1.

11. L. Hallberg et al., "Iron Absorption from Southeast Asian Diets," *American Journal of Clinical Nutrition* 30 (1977): 539–48.

12. Walter Gratzer, *Terrors of the Table: The Curious History of Nutrition* (Oxford: OUP, 2005), 246.

AUSTEN EATS: BREAD

1. Mireille Guiliano, *French Women Don't Get Fat: The Secrets of Eating for Pleasure* (New York: Knopf, 2005), 254.

2. Charles P. Moritz, *Travels, Chiefly on Foot, Through Several Parts of England, in 1782* (London: G.G. and J. Robinson, 1797), 27.

3. Kate Fox, *Watching the English: The Hidden Rules of English Behavior*, rev. ed. (London: Hodder and Stoughton, 2014), 444.

4. A. B. Geier et al., "Unit Bias: A New Heuristic That Helps Explain the Effect of Portion Size on Food Intake," *Psychological Science* 17 (2006): 521–25.

5. Bill Bryson, *At Home: A Short History of Private Life* (New York: Anchor Book, 2011), 80–81.

6. Tobias Smollett, *Humphry Clinker*, edited by Shaun Regan (reprint; New York: Penguin, 2008), 136.

7. Stephen Yafa, *Grain of Truth: The Real Case for and Against Wheat and Gluten* (New York: Avery, 2015), 18, 99.

8. Ibid., 59.

9. Butylated Hydroxyanisole (BHA), CAS No. 25013-16-5, *Report on Carcinogens*, 14th ed., National Institutes of Health. Available at https://ntp.niehs.nih.gov/pubhealth/roc/index-1.html

10. Janet Macdonald, *Feeding Nelson's Navy: The True Story of Food at Sea in the Georgian Era* (London: Chatham, 2004), 17.

11. Carlo G. Rizzello et al., "Highly Efficient Gluten Degradation by Lactobacilli and Fungal Proteases During Food Processing: New Perspectives for Celiac Disease," *Applied and Environmental Microbiology* 73 (2007): 4499–4507.

3. THE PEMBERLEY MEAL PLAN

1. Maggie Lane, *Jane Austen and Food* (London: Hambledon, 1995), 25–27.

2. Michael Mosley and Mimi Spencer, *The Fast Diet: Lose Weight, Stay Healthy, and Live Longer with the Simple Secret of Intermittent Fasting* (New York: Atria, 2013),

24–25; "Easy Health Hack: A Late Breakfast is Michael Mosley's Secret Weapon" by Bonnie Bayley, *SBS* (AU.), September 22, 2016. Available at https://www.sbs.com.au /food/article/2016/09/20/easy-health-hack-late-breakfast -michael-mosleys-secret-weapon.

3. "Early Morning is Actually the Worst Time to Drink Coffee" by Kia Kokalitcheva, *Time*, June 1, 2015. Available at http:// time.com/3903826/coffee-early-morning-worst-time/.

4. Kim Wilson, *Tea with Jane Austen* (Madison, WI: Jones Books, 2004), 2–4.

5. Roy and Lesley Adkins, *Jane Austen's England* (New York: Viking, 2013), 113.

6. Carolly Erickson, *Our Tempestuous Day: A History of Regency England* (New York: William Morrow, 1986), 221.

7. Colin Spencer, *British Food: An Extraordinary Thousand Years of History*, quoting *Jane Eyre* and *Wuthering Heights* (New York: Columbia University Press, 2002), 258.

8. "Impact of Circadian Misalignment on Energy Metabolism During Simulated Nightshift Work," *Proceedings of the National Academy of Sciences* 111 (2014): 17302–17307.

9. John Ashton, *Social England Under the Regency*, vol. 1 (London: Ward and Downey, 1890) 302–303.

10. "Timing of Serving Dessert but Not Portion Size Affects Young Children's Intake at Lunchtime," *Appetite* 68 (2013): 158–63.

11. A. Roger Ekirch, *At Day's Close: Night in Times Past*, quoting Stephen Bradwell (New York: Norton, 2005), 271.

12. Thomas Preston, *Dictionary of English Proverbs and Proverbial Phrases* (1880).

13. "How Soup Can Help You Lose Weight" by Jack Challoner, *BBC News*, May 26, 2009. Available at http://news.bbc .co.uk/2/hi/uk_news/magazine/8068733.stm.

14. Walter Gratzer, *Terrors of the Table: The Curious History of Nutrition* (Oxford: OUP, 2005), 229.

15. Spencer, *British Food*, quoting Samuel Johnson, 256.

16. Nina Teicholz, *The Big Fat Surprise: Why Butter, Meat, and Cheese Belong in a Healthy Diet* (New York: Simon and Schuster, 2014), 296; Gratzer, *Terrors of the Table*, 228.

17. John Durant, *The Paleo Manifesto: Ancient Wisdom for Lifelong Health* (New York: Harmony, 2013), 134.

AUSTEN EATS: SUGAR

1. A rough percentage based on sugar consumption figures per capita in late eighteenth-century England and modern America. See notes 3 and 4 below.

2. Maggie Lane, *Jane Austen and Food* (London: Hambledon, 1995), 17.

3. James Walvin, *Fruits of Empire: Exotic Produce and British Taste* (New York: New York University Press, 1997), 119.

4. "Is Sugar Toxic?" by Gary Taubes, *New York Times Magazine*, April 13, 2011. Available at https://www.nytimes.com /2011/04/17/magazine/mag-17Sugar-t.html.

5. R. K. Johnson et al., "Dietary Sugars Intake and Cardiovascular Health: A Scientific Statement from the American Heart Association," *Circulation* 120 (2009): 1011–1020.

6. John Durant, *The Paleo Manifesto: Ancient Wisdom for Lifelong Health* (New York: Harmony, 2013), 134, and previous note 4.

7. Walter Gratzer, *Terrors of the Table: The Curious History of Nutrition* (Oxford: Oxford University Press, 2005), 212.

8. P. M. Wise et al., "Reduced Dietary Intake of Simple Sugars Alters Perceived Sweet Taste Intensity but Not Perceived Pleasantness," *American Journal of Clinical Nutrition* 103 (2016): 50–60.

9. Robert H. Lustig, *Fat Chance: Beating the Odds Against Sugar, Processed Food, Obesity, and Disease* (New York: Hudson Street Press, 2012), 234.

10. Attested by the meticulous meal records of Parson Woodforde (1740–1803), whose diaries provide some of the best
peeks into middle-class eating habits of the era.

11. Jotham Suez et al., "Artificial Sweeteners Induce Glucose
Intolerance by Altering the Gut Microbiota," *Nature* 514
(2014): 181–86.

4. DRINKS WITH JANE

1. Kim Wilson, *Tea with Jane Austen* (Madison, WI: Jones
Books, 2004), 56.

2. Markman Ellis, Richard Coulton, and Matthew Mauger,
Empire of Tea: The Asian Leaf that Conquered the World,
quoting Samuel Tissot (London: Reaktion, 2015), 106.

3. 350 AD marks the first official mention of tea in a Chinese
dictionary by scholar Kuo Po.

4. Mary Lou Heiss and Robert J. Heiss, *The Story of Tea: A
Cultural History and Drinking Guide* (Berkeley: Ten Speed
Press, 2007), 7.

5. Mike Ukra, *The Ultimate Tea Diet* (New York: Collins),
40–42.

6. "The Truth About Alcohol," directed by David Briggs (2016;
BBC One), television.

7. "Black Tea Alters Gut Microbiome in Anti-Obesogenic
Ways" by Christopher Bergland, *Psychology Today*,
October 4, 2017. Available at http://www.psychologytoday
.com/us/blog/the-athletes-way/201710/black-tea-alters
-gut-microbiome-in-anti-obesogenic-ways.

8. Roy Moxham, *Tea: Addiction, Exploitation, and Empire*,
quoting Samuel Johnson (New York: Carroll and Graf,
2003), 34.

9. A. C. Nobre et al., "L-theanine, a Natural Constituent in
Tea, and Its Effect on Mental State," *Asia Pacific Journal of
Clinical Nutrition* 17 (2008): 167–68.

10. K. Lu et al., "The Acute Effects of L-theanine in Comparison with Alprazolam on Anticipatory Anxiety in Humans," *Human Psychopharmacology* 19 (2004): 457–65.

11. Beatrice Hohenegger, *Liquid Jade: The Story of Tea from East to West*, quoting Lu T-ung (New York: St. Martin's Press, 2006), 20.

12. Frederick A. Pottle ed., *Boswell's London Journal 1762-1763*, 2nd ed. (New Haven: Yale University Press, 2004), 189.

13. Wilson, *Tea with Jane Austen*, 50.

14. "A Very British Response to Terror" by Rossalyn Warren, *New York Times*, June 4, 2017. Available at https://www.nytimes.com/2017/06/04/opinion/london-bridge-terrorist-attack.html.

15. Sarah Rose, *For All the Tea in China: How England Stole the World's Favorite Drink and Changed History* (New York: Viking, 2010), 164.

16. Tobias Smollett, *Humphry Clinker*, edited by Shaun Regan (reprint; New York: Penguin, 2008), 135.

17. "Tea 'Healthier' Drink than Water," *BBC News*, August 24, 2006. Available at http://news.bbc.co.uk/2/hi/health/5281046.stm.

18. Ibid.

19. E. J. Gardner et al., "Black Tea—Helpful or Harmful? A Review of the Evidence," *European Journal of Clinical Nutrition* 61 (2007): 3–18.

20. M. Lorenz et al., "Addition of Milk Prevents Vascular Protective Effects of Tea," *European Heart Journal* 28 (2007): 219–23.

21. A.G. Sharper, "British Regional Heart Study: Cardiovascular Mortality and Water Quality," *Journal of Environmental Pathology and Toxicology* 3 (1980): 89–111.

22. "Magnesium is Essential to Your Health, But Many People Don't Get Enough of It" by Consumer Report,

Washington Post, June 10, 2017. Available at https://
www.washingtonpost.com/national/health-science
/magnesium-is-essential-to-your-health-but-many-people
-dont-get-enough-of-it/2017/06/09/77bc35b4-2515-11e7
-bb9d-8cd6118e1409_story.html?utm_term=.ec3db34f7288.

23. "The Best of Bath, England" by Joanne Shurvell, *Forbes*,
July 18, 2016. Available at https://www.forbes.com/sites
/joanneshurvell/2016/07/18/the-best-of-bath-england/.

24. "Soda Stats: How Those Empty Calories Add Up" by Yunji de
Neis and Hanna Siegel, *ABC News*, April 21, 2010. Available
at http://abcnews.go.com/WN/soda-statistics-empty-calories
-add/story?id=10303246.

25. Bharat Tandon ed., *Emma: An Annotated Edition*, quoting
A. F. M. Willich and William Nisbet (Cambridge: Harvard
University Press, 2012), 382–83.

26. Stephen Le, *100 Million Years of Food: What Our Ancestors
Ate and Why It Matters Today* (New York: Picador, 2016),
105.

27. Liza Picard, *Dr. Johnson's London*, quoting *The Ladies
Magazine* [July 1750] (New York: St. Martin's Press, 2000),
124.

28. Maggie Lane, *Jane Austen and Food* (London: Hambledon,
1995), 45–46.

29. Richard B. Schwartz, *Daily Life in Johnson's London* (Madison, WI: University of Wisconsin Press, 1983), 74.

30. Roy Porter, *Flesh in the Age of Reason: The Modern Foundations of Body and Soul*, quoting Sylas Neville (New York:
Norton, 2003), 236.

31. Z. Zupan et al., "Wine Glass Size in England from 1700 to
2017: A Measure of Our Time," *British Medical Journal* 359
(2017).

32. "Wine Drinkers Often Overpour, Study Says" by Sharyn
Jackson, *USA Today*, September 30, 2013. Available at
https://www.usatoday.com/story/news/nation/2013/09/30
/wine-serving-size-too-much/2895661/.

NOTES

AUSTEN EATS: MEAT

1. Emma Thompson, *The Sense and Sensibility Screenplay and Diaries* (New York: Newmarket Press, 1995), 103.

2. Sandie Byrne, *Jane Austen's Possessions and Dispossessions* (London: Palgrave Macmillan, 2014), 18.

3. Hannah Glasse, *The Art of Cookery Made Plain and Easy* (1747 reprint, New York: Dover Publications, 2015), 278.

4. C. Anne Wilson, *Food and Drink in Britain: From the Stone Age to the 19th Century*, quoting F. M. Misson, *Memoirs* [1719] (Chicago: Academy Chicago Publishers, 1991), 97.

5. Charles Lamb, ed. Adam Phillips, *Selected Prose* (New York: Penguin, 1985), 165.

6. R. G. Jensen, "The Lipids in Human Milk," *Lipids* 34 (1999): 40.

7. "Julia Child: What I've Learned" by Mike Sager, *Esquire*, June 2000, 121.

8. Nina Teicholz, *The Big Fat Surprise: Why Butter, Meat and Cheese Belong in a Healthy Diet* (New York: Simon and Schuster, 2014), 311.

9. Ibid., 11–12.

10. P. W. Siri-Tarino et al., "Meta-analysis of Prospective Cohort Studies Evaluating the Association of Saturated Fat with Cardiovascular Disease," *American Journal of Clinical Nutrition* 91 (2010): 535–46.

11. Barbara V. Howard et al., "Low-Fat Dietary Pattern and Weight Change Over 7 Years: The Women's Health Initiative Dietary Modification Trial," *Journal of the American Medical Association* 295 (2006): 39–49; Barbara V. Howard et al., "Low-Fat Dietary Pattern and Risk of Cardiovascular Disease: The Women's Health Initiative Randomized Controlled Dietary Modification Trial," *Journal of the American Medical Association* 295 (2006): 655–56.

12. Lucy Worsley, *If Walls Could Talk: An Intimate History of the Home*, quoting Thomas Elyot, *Castell of Health* [1536] (New York: Walker and Company, 2011), 287.

13. Roy Porter, *The Greatest Benefit to Mankind: A Medical History of Humanity from Antiquity to the Present* (New York: Norton, 1997), 281.

14. Roy Porter and G. S. Rousseau, *Gout: The Patrician Malady* (New Haven: Yale University Press, 2000), 3, 49.

15. Vilhjalmur Stefansson, *The Fat of the Land*, engl. ed. of *Not By Bread Alone* (1946, reprint; New York: Macmillan, 1956), xvi.

16. John Ashton, *Social England Under the Regency*, 2 vols. (London: Ward and Downey, 1890), 302–303.

17. Jennifer McLagan, *Fat: An Appreciation of a Misunderstood Ingredient* (Berkeley: Ten Speed Press, 2008), 201.

18. Cynthia A. Daley et al., "A Review of Fatty Acid Profiles and Antioxidant Content in Grass-Fed and Grain-Fed Beef," *Nutrition Journal* 9 (2010): 10.

19. M. A. Crawford et al., "Comparative Studies on Fatty Acid Composition of Wild and Domestic Meats," *International Journal of Biochemistry* 1 (1970): 295–305.

20. Tanya Blasbalg et al., "Changes in Consumption of Omega-3 and Omega-6 Fatty Acids in the United States During the 20th Century," *American Journal of Clinical Nutrition* 93 (2011): 950–62.

21. "Which Oils are Best to Cook With?" by Michael Mosley, *BBC*, July 28, 2015. Available at http://www.bbc.com/news/magazine-33675975.

5. WALK LIKE AN ELIZABETH

1. Katherine Schreiber and Heather A. Hausenblas, *The Truth About Exercise Addiction: Understanding the Dark Side of Thinspiration* (Lanham, MD: Rowman and Littlefield, 2015), 61.

2. Lucy Worsley, *Jane Austen at Home: A Biography*, quoting Edmund Burke (New York: St. Martin's Press, 2017), 53.

3. Bharat Tandon, ed., *Emma: An Annotated Edition*, quoting Mary Wollstonecraft (Cambridge: Harvard University Press, 2012), 333.

4. Roy Porter, *Flesh in the Age of Reason: The Modern Foundations of Body and Soul* (New York: Norton, 2003), 51.

5. Ibid., quoting Joseph Addison, 119.

6. J. N. Morris et al., "Coronary Heart Disease and Physical Activity of Work," *Lancet* 265 (1953): 1053–1057.

7. Carl J. Lavie with Kristin Loberg, *The Obesity Paradox: When Thinner Means Sicker and Heavier Means Healthier* (New York: Hudson Street Press, 2014), 65–66.

8. Roy and Lesley Adkins, *Jane Austen's England*, quoting James Woodforde (New York: Viking, 2013), 239.

9. Valerie Grosvenor Myer, *Jane Austen, Obstinate Heart: A Biography* (New York: Arcade, 1997), 104.

10. Based on the calculation that the average American walks 2.5 miles a day with a typical walking speed of about 3 miles per hour. Sources: Dan Rubinstein, *Born to Walk: The Transformative Power of a Pedestrian Act* (Ontario, ECW Press, 2015), 10; Stephen Le, *100 Million Years of Food: What Our Ancestors Ate and Why It Matters Today* (New York: Picador, 2016), 163.

11. Liza Picard, *Dr. Johnson's London*, quoting Dr. George Cheyne (New York: St. Martin's Press, 2000), 161.

12. Dan Rubinstein, *Born to Walk: The Transformative Power of a Pedestrian Act*, quoting Louis Philippe (Ontario: ECW Press, 2015), 10.

13. "Why Walking," American Heart Association, July 26, 2016. Available at http://www.heart.org/HEARTORG/HealthyLiving/PhysicalActivity/Walking/Why-Walking_UCM_461770_Article.jsp?appName=WebApp#.Ws5DJmz7lZU.

14. David R. Basset et al., "Physical Activity in an Old Order Amish Community," *Medicine and Science in Sports and Exercise* 36 (2004): 79–85; Stephen Le, *100 Million Years of Food: What Our Ancestors Ate and Why It Matters Today* (New York: Picador, 2016), 213.

15. Eva M. Selhub and Alan C. Logan, *Your Brain on Nature: The Science of Nature's Influence on Your Health, Happiness, and Vitality* (Ontario: Collins, 2014), 121.

16. Carolina O. C. Werle et al., "Is It Fun or Exercise? The Framing of Physical Activity Biases Subsequent Snacking," *Marketing Letters* (May 15, 2014).

17. James Blumenthal et al., "Exercise Treatment for Major Depression: Maintenance of Therapeutic Benefit at 10 Months," *Psychosomatic Medicine* 62 (2000): 633–38.

18. D. W. Dunstan et al., "Breaking Up Prolonged Sitting Reduces Postprandial Glucose and Insulin Responses," *Diabetes Care* 35 (2012): 976–83.

19. Selub and Logan, *Your Brain on Nature*, 116–19.

20. H. R. Patil et al., "Cardiovascular Damage Resulting from Chronic Excessive Endurance Exercise," *Missouri Medicine* 109 (2012): 312–21.

21. Hippocrates, *Hippocratic Writings* (Chicago: Encyclopedia Britannica, 1955).

22. Emma Thompson, *The Sense and Sensibility Screenplay and Diaries*, also quoting Jane Gibson (New York: New Market Press, 1995), 213.

23. Francois Nivelon, *The Rudiments of Genteel Behavior* (London: 1737).

24. Thompson, *Sense and Sensibility Screenplay*, 212.

25. James Edward Austen-Leigh, *A Memoir of Jane Austen*, 2nd ed. (London: R. Bentley and Son, 1871), 30–31.

26. D. R. Carney et al., "Power Posing: Brief Nonverbal Displays Affect Neuroendocrine Levels and Risk Tolerance," *Psychological Science* 21 (2010): 1363–68; Erik Peper et

al., "Increase or Decrease Depression—How Body Postures Influence Your Energy Levels," *Biofeedback* 40 (2012): 126–30.

27. M. Zentner et al., "Rhythmic Engagement with Music in Infancy," *Proceedings of the National Academy of Sciences* 107 (2010): 5768–5773.

28. Richard Louv, *The Nature Principle: Human Restoration and the End of Nature-Deficit Disorder*, quoting *The English Gardener* [1670] (Chapel Hill, NC: Algonquin Books, 2011), 46.

29. Lucy Worsley, *Jane Austen at Home: A Biography*, quoting Cassandra Austen (New York: St. Martin's Press, 2017), 17.

30. Selub and Logan, *Your Brain on Nature*, 156–58.

AUSTEN EATS: CARBS

1. E. L. McAdam Jr. and George Milne, ed., *Johnson's Dictionary: A Modern Selection,* (New York: Modern Library, 1963), 268.

2. Jean Anthelme Brillat-Savarin, *The Physiology of Taste*, translated by M. F. K. Fisher (New York: Counterpoint Press, 1971), 237–51.

3. *The Complete Farmer*, 5th ed. (London, 1807).

4. Leo Tolstoy, *Anna Karenina*, translated by Constance Garnett (New York: Modern Library Classics, 2000), 200.

6. "A TASTE FOR NATURE"

1. The "biophilia hypothesis" (human's innate need for nature) was popularized by Harvard biologist Edward O. Wilson in his book *Biophilia* (Harvard University Press, 1984).

2. Shawn Stevenson, *Sleep Smarter: 21 Essential Strategies to Sleep Your Way to a Better Body, Better Health, and Bigger Success* (New York: Rodale, 2016), 9.

3. Ibid, 12–14.

NOTES

4. Jeffrey Rossman, *The Mind-Body Mood Solution: The Breakthrough Drug-Free Program for Lasting Relief from Depression* (New York: Rodale, 2011), 93.

5. J. J. Alvarsson et al., "Stress Recovery During Exposure to Nature Sound and Environmental Noise," *International Journal of Environmental Research and Public Health* 7 (2010): 1036–1046.

6. K. Kaida, "Self-Awakening Prevents Acute Rise in Blood Pressure and Heart Rate at the Time of Awakening in Elderly People," *Industrial Health* 43 (2005): 179–85.

7. Maurine Witte, "Lord David Cecil," *Persuasions* [a publication of the Jane Austen Society of North America] 4 (1982): 6–7.

8. Emma Thompson, *The Sense and Sensibility Screenplay and Diaries* (New York: New Market Press, 1995), 84.

9. G. Lambert et al., "Effect of Sunlight and Season on Serotonin Turnover in the Brain," *The Lancet* 360 (2002): 1840–1842.

10. R. S. Ulrich, "View Through Window May Influence Recovery from Surgery," *Science* 224 (1984): 420–21.

11. K. M. Hanson, "Sunscreen Enhancement of UV-Induced Reactive Oxygen Species in the Skin," *Free Radical Biology and Medicine* 41 (2006): 1205–1212.

12. "Can Cheap Sunglasses Be Bad for Your Eyes?" by Tiffany Sharples, *Time*, August 4, 2009. Available at http://healthland.time.com/2009/08/04/can-cheap-sunglasses-be-bad-for-your-eyes/.

13. Roy and Lesley Adkins, *Jane Austen's England* (New York: Viking, 2013), 96.

14. Z. Bakò-Birò et al., "Effects of Pollution from Personal Computers on Perceived Air Quality, SBS Symptoms and Productivity in Offices," *Indoor Air* 14 (2004): 178–87.

15. Eva M. Selhub and Alan C. Logan, *Your Brain on Nature: The Science of Nature's Influence on Your Health, Happiness, and Vitality* (Ontario: Collins, 2012), 98.

16. Ibid., 99.

17. C. A. Gilkeson et al., "Measurement of Ventilation and Airborne Infection Risk in Large Naturally Ventilated Hospital Wards," *Building and Environment* 65 (2013): 35–48.

18. "Top Five Health Problems Associated with Air Conditioning" by Nicole Bogart, *Global News*, June 20, 2012. Available at https://globalnews.ca/news/258330/top-5-health-problems -associated-with-air-conditioning/.

19. "Is New-Car Smell Bad for Your Health?" by Jim Travers, *BBC*, March 15, 2016. Available at http://www.bbc.com/autos /story/20160315-is-new-car-smell-bad-for-your-health.

20. Yoshifumi Miyazaki et al., "Phytoncides (wood essential oils) Induce Human Natural Killer Cell Activity," *Immunopharmacology and Immunotoxicology* 28 (2006): 313–33.

21. Richard Louv, *The Nature Principle: Human Restoration and the End of Nature-Deficit Disorder* (Chapel Hill, NC: Algonquin Books, 2011). 30, 60.22; Lucy Worsley, *Jane Austen at Home: A Biography* (New York: St. Martin's Press, 2017), 112.

23. Selhub and Logan, *Your Brain on Nature*, 90.

24. Louv, *The Nature Principle*, 178.

25. Selhub and Logan, *Your Brain on Nature*, 90.

26. A. M. Change, "Evening Use of Light-Emitting eReaders Negatively Affects Sleep, Circadian Timing, and Next Morning Alertness," *Proceedings of the National Academy of Sciences* 112 (2015): 1232–1237.

27. Selhub and Logan, *Your Brain on Nature*, 90.

28. "Blue Light Has a Dark Side," *Harvard Health Letter*, May 2012. Available at https://www.health.harvard.edu /staying-healthy/blue-light-has-a-dark-side.

29. Stevenson, *Sleep Smarter*, 75.

30. Selhub and Logan, *Your Brain on Nature*, 28.

NOTES

AUSTEN EATS: GARDEN STUFF

1. Gyles Brandreth, ed., *Oxford Dictionary of Humorous Quotations* (Oxford: OUP, 2013), 125.

2. Lucy Worsley, *At Home with Jane Austen: A Biography* (New York: St. Martin's Press, 2017), 193.

3. Tobias Smollett, *Humphry Clinker*, edited by Shaun Regan (reprint; New York: Penguin, 2008), 133–34.

4. Gilbert White, *The Natural History and Antiquities of Selborne* (London: Benjamin White and Son, 1789); reprint (London: Macmillan, 1900), 190.

5. Louis Simond, *Journal of a Tour and Residence in Great Britain*, 2 vols. (Edinburgh: 1815), i. 57.

6. Jack Ayres, ed., *Paupers and Pig Killers: The Diary of William Holland, a Somerset Parson* (Gloucester: Allan Sutton, 1984), 38.

7. Stephen Le, *100 Million Years of Food: What Our Ancestors Ate and Why It Matters Today* (New York: Picador, 2016), 89.

8. Center for Food Safety and Applied Nutrition, *The Bad Bug Book: Foodborne Pathogenic Microorganisms and Natural Toxins Handbook* (Washington: U.S. Food and Drug Administration, 1992), 254.

9. Colin Spencer, *British Food: An Extraordinary Thousand Years of History* (New York: Columbia University Press, 2002), 234.

10. "Fact or Fiction: Raw Veggies are Healthier Than Cooked Ones" by Sushma Subramanian, *Scientific American*, March 31, 2009. Available at https:/www.scientificamerican .com/article/raw-veggies-are-healthier/.

11. In 1747, James Lind, a physician in the Royal Navy, conducted history's first clinical trial into curing scurvy with citrus fruits, publishing his findings in *A Treatise of the Scurvy* (1753).

12. Maggie Lane, *Jane Austen and Food* (London: Hambledon, 1995), 64.

13. "Got Fat? You need it to reap cancer-prevention benefits of vegetables, says Iowa State University Professor," *Iowa State University News Service*, July 22, 2002. Available at https://www.news.iastate.edu/news/2004/jul/whitebetac .shtml.

7. "HEALTH AND HAPPINESS"

1. Jo Marchant, *Cure: A Journey into the Science of Mind Over Body* (New York: Crown, 2016), xiv.

2. Roy Porter, *Flesh in the Age of Reason: The Modern Foundations of Body and Soul*, quoting William Godwin (New York: Norton, 2003), 427.

3. Marchant, *Cure*, xiv.

4. Porter, *Flesh in the Age of Reason*, 427.

5. "How Happiness Boosts the Immune System," by Jo Marchant, *Scientific American*, November 27, 2013. Available at https://www.scientificamerican.com/article/how-happiness -boosts-the-immune-system/.

6. William James, *The Principles of Psychology* vol. 1 (New York: Henry Holt, 1890), 402.

7. B. J. Bushman, "Does Venting Anger Feed or Extinguish the Flame? Catharsis, Rumination, Distraction, Anger, and Aggressive Responding," *Personality and Social Psychology Bulletin* 28 (2002): 724–31.

8. Jonathan Rose, *The Literary Churchill: Author, Reader, Actor*, quoting Winston Churchill (New Haven: Yale University Press, 2014), 369.

9. Margaret Smith, ed., *The Letters of Charlotte Brontë, Volume Two 1848–1851* (Oxford: Clarendon Press, 2000), 10.

10. Lucy Worsley, *Jane Austen at Home: A Biography* (New York: St. Martin's Press, 2017), 102.

NOTES

11. Ibid., quoting *Letter to the Women of England on the Injustice of Mental Subordination* [1799], 103.

12. Traci Mann, *Secrets from the Eating Lab: The Science of Weight Loss, the Myth of Willpower, and Why You Should Never Diet Again* (New York: Harper Wave, 2015), 58.

13. Marchant, *Cure*, 136–37.

14. J. P. Boone, "Evaluating the Impact of Stress on Systemic Disease: the MOST Protocol in Primary Care," *Journal of the American Osteopathic Association* 103 (2003): 239–46.

15. E. S. Epel et al., "Accelerated Telomere Shortening in Response to Life Stress," *Proceedings of the National Academy of Sciences* 101 (2004): 17312–17315.

16. David Nokes, *Jane Austen: A Life* (Berkley: University of California Press, 1997), 353.

17. Richard Arthur Austen-Leigh, *Austen Papers 1704–1856*, quoting Elizabeth de Feuillide [May 3, 1797] (Colchester: 1942), 158–60; James Edward Austen-Leigh, *A Memoir of Jane Austen*, 2nd ed. (London: Richard Bentley and Son, 1871), 16.

18. M. G. Marmot et al., "Health Inequalities Among British Civil Servants: The Whitehall II Study," *Lancet* 337 (1991): 1393–1397.

19. Virginia Woolf, *The Common Reader* (New York: Harcourt, 1925), 139.

20. Norman Cousins, "Anatomy of an Illness (as Perceived by the Patient)," *New England Journal of Medicine* 295 (1976): 1458–1463.

21. "Smiling Can Trick Your Brain into Happiness—and Boost Your Health" by Nicole Spector, *NBC News*, November 28, 2017. Available at https://www.nbcnews.com/better/health/smiling-can-trick-your-brain-happiness-boost-your-health-ncna822591.

22. P. Sasannejad, "Lavender Essential Oil in the Treatment of Migraine Headache: a Placebo-Controlled Clinical Trial," *European Neurology* 67 (2012): 284–91.

23. *Sense and Sensibility*, directed by John Alexander (2008; BBC Video), DVD.

24. C. Stout et al., "Unusually Low Incidence of Death from Myocardial Infarction: Study of an Italian-American Community in Pennsylvania," *Journal of the American Medical Association* 188 (1964): 845–49; Anne Harrington, *The Cure Within: A History of Mind-Body Medicine* (New York: Norton, 2008), 177–79.

25. Harrington, *The Cure Within,* 176.

26. "Why Silence Is Good for Your Brain" by Carolyn Gregoire, *Huffington Post*, March 5, 2016. Available at https://www.huffingtonpost.com/entry/silence-brain-benefits_us_56d83967e4b0000de4037004.

27. L. Bernardi et al., "Cardiovascular, Cerebrovascular, and Respiratory Changes Induced by Different Types of Music in Musicians and Non-Musicians: The Importance of Silence," *Heart* 92 (2006): 445–52.

28. "Love Letters and Kindness May Improve Mental Health" by Lorna Stewart, *BBC News*, March 23, 2013. Available at http://www.bbc.com/news/health-21900202.